AF674706

Atlas of Hematology

Atlas of Hematology

Renu Saxena MBBS, MD (Pathology)
Professor and Head
Department of Hematology
All India Institute of Medical Sciences (AIIMS)
Ansari Nagar, New Delhi

HP Pati MBBS, MD (Pathology)
Professor
Department of Hematology
All India Institute of Medical Sciences (AIIMS)
Ansari Nagar, New Delhi

M Mahapatra MBBS, MD (Internal Medicine)
Additional Professor
Department of Hematology
All India Institute of Medical Sciences (AIIMS)
Ansari Nagar, New Delhi

JAYPEE BROTHERS MEDICAL PUBLISHERS (P) LTD

New Delhi • Panama City • London

Jaypee Brothers Medical Publishers (P) Ltd.

Headquarter

Jaypee Brothers Medical Publishers (P) Ltd
4838/24, Ansari Road, Daryaganj
New Delhi 110 002, India
Phone: +91-11-43574357
Fax: +91-11-43574314
Email: jaypee@jaypeebrothers.com

Overseas Offices

J.P. Medical Ltd.,
83 Victoria Street London
SW1H 0HW (UK)
Phone: +44-2031708910
Fax: +02-03-0086180
Email: info@jpmedpub.com

Jaypee-Highlights Medical Publishers Inc.
City of Knowledge, Bld. 237, Clayton
Panama City, Panama
Phone: 507-317-0160
Fax: +50-73-010499
Email: cservice@jphmedical.com

Website: www.jaypeebrothers.com
Website: www.jaypeedigital.com

© 2012, Jaypee Brothers Medical Publishers

Inquiries for bulk sales may be solicited at: jaypee@jaypeebrothers.com

This book has been published in good faith that the contents provided by the authors contained herein are original, and is intended for educational purposes only. While every effort is made to ensure a accuracy of information, the publisher and the authors specifically disclaim any damage, liability, or loss incurred, directly or indirectly, from the use or application of any of the contents of this work. If not specifically stated, all figures and tables are courtesy of the authors. Where appropriate, the readers should consult with a specialist or contact the manufacturer of the drug or device.

Publisher: Jitendar P Vij

Publishing Director: Tarun Duneja

Cover Design: Seema Dogra

Atlas of Hematology

First Edition: **2012**

ISBN 978-93-5025-508-7

Printed at Replika Press Pvt. Ltd.

Preface

There has been a long felt need for an Atlas of Hematology. With this in mind, our endeavor in this atlas was to give representative clinical photographs and microphotographs of some of the commonly seen hematological disorders. This book is likely to be helpful to pediatricians, internists and pathologists practicing hematology, undergraduates and postgraduates of pediatrics, medicine and pathology, especially in centers where many of these lesions are not commonly seen. We hope this book will be useful to the readers.

Renu Saxena
HP Pati
M Mahapatra

Acknowledgments

We would like to acknowledge Dr Narender Tejwani DM, Resident, Department of Hematopathology, AIIMS for meticulous proofreading and Mr Harinder Kumar for secretarial help.

Contents

Chapter One

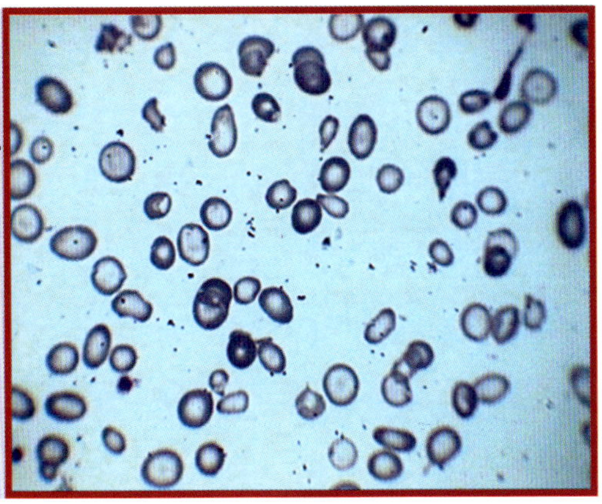

Chapter Two

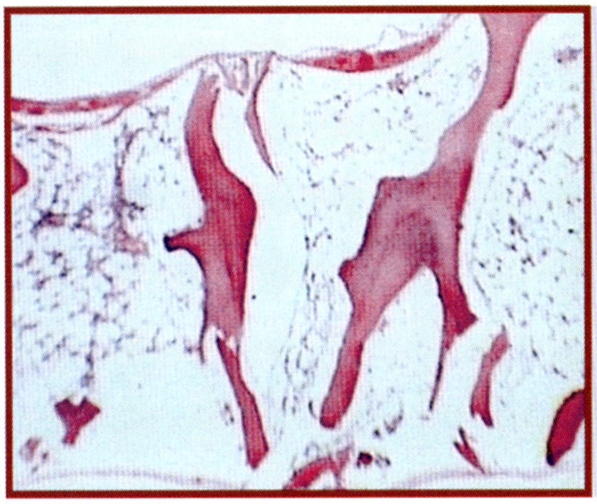

Chapter Three

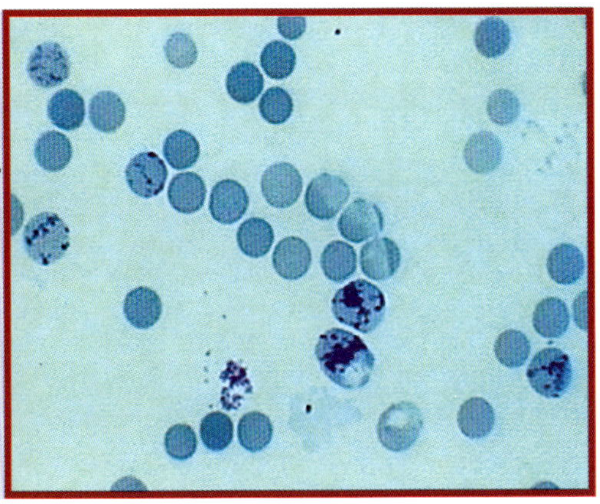

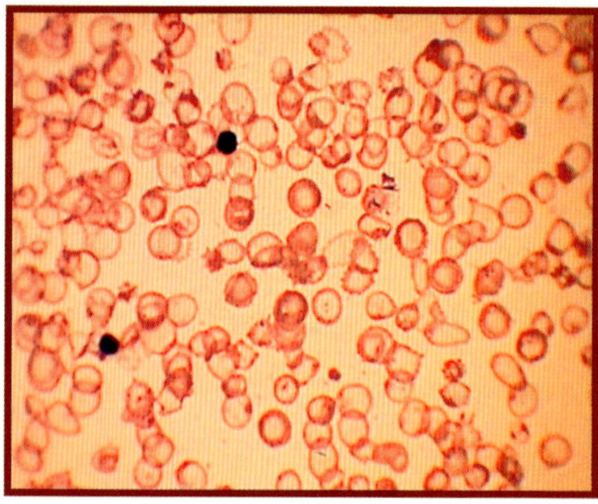

Chapter Four

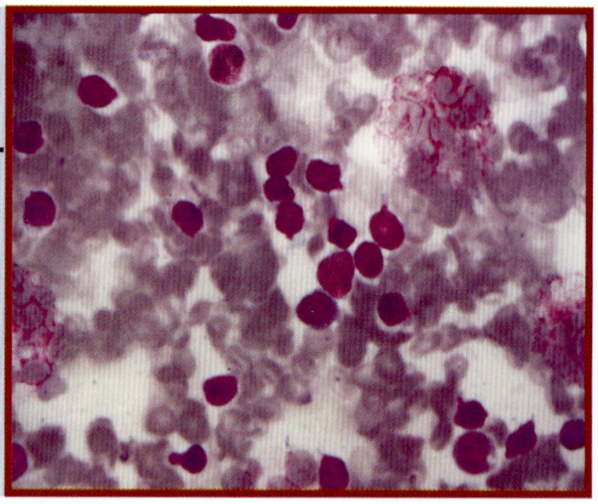

Chapter Five

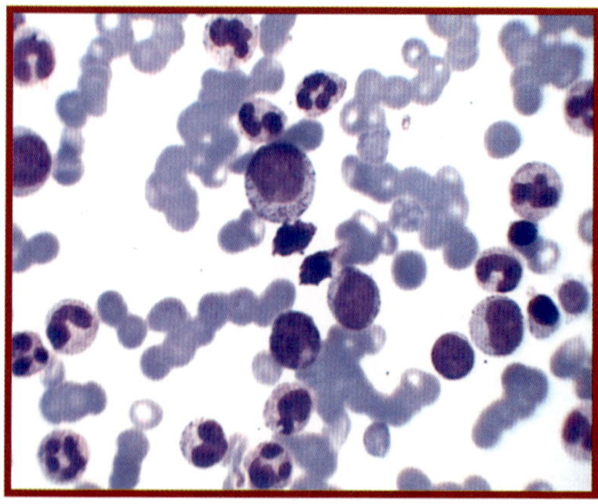

Chapter Six

Chapter Seven

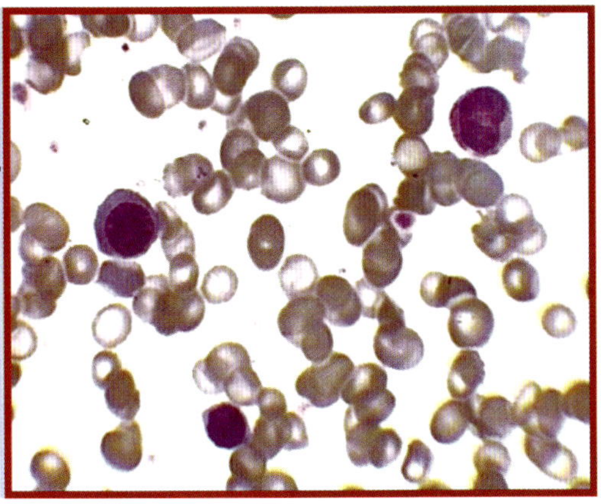

Myelofibrosis 84

Plasma Cell Dyscrasias 88

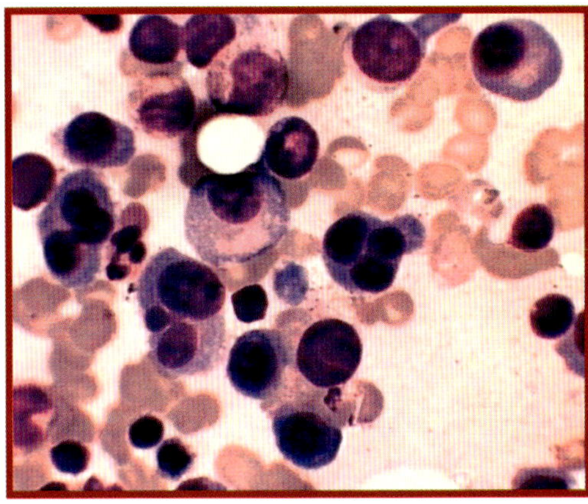

Chapter Eight

Chapter Nine

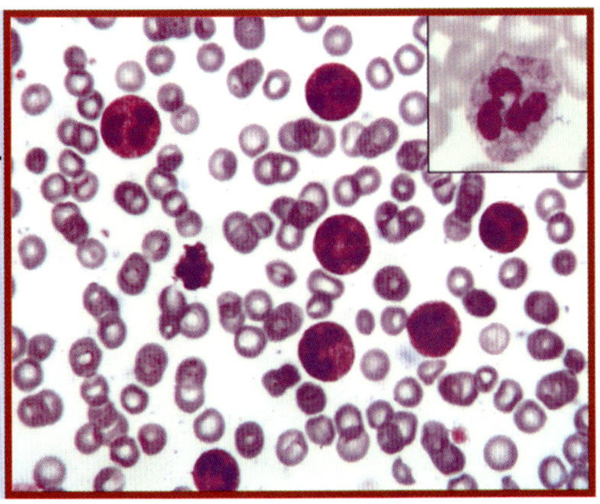

Infections 94

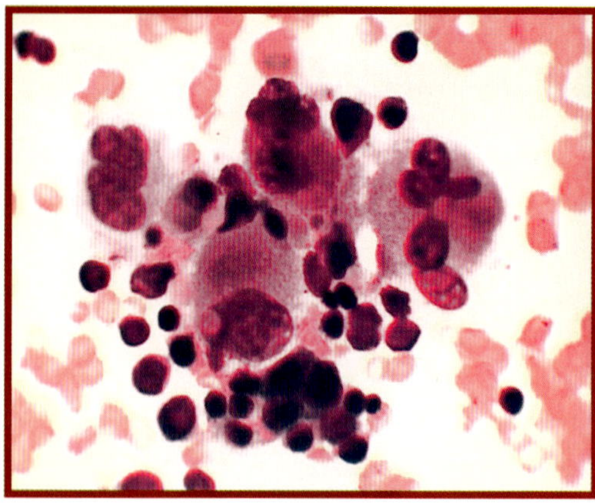

Chapter Ten

CHAPTER 1

Anemias

CHAPTER OVERVIEW

- Investigation
- Hypochromic microcytic anemia
- Sideroblastic anemia
- Macrocytic anemia
- Dimorphic anemia
- Myelodysplastic syndrome (MDS)
- Normocytic normochromic anemia

Anemia is one of the most common clinical presentation. Amongst these, anemia due to nutrient deficiency such as iron, vitamin B_{12} or folic acid are very common. Folate deficiency is much more common than B_{12} deficiency since liver stores for vitamin B_{12} last for five to six years whereas stores for folic acid last for three to four months. Iron deficiency anemia, particularly mild to moderate, may cause a problem in differential diagnosis from other hypochromic anemias like beta thalassemia trait, alpha thalassemia trait, Hb E disease, sideroblastic anemia or anemia of chronic disorder.

INVESTIGATION

For diagnosis of anemia, the following preliminary investigations are most important:

- Hemoglobin, hematocrit (PCV)
- Red cell indices: MCV, MCH, MCHC, RDW (with automated cell counters)
- Reticulocyte count

Based on these tests, anemia subtypes can be made, which helps in reaching a diagnosis (Fig. 1.1).

HYPOCHROMIC MICROCYTIC ANEMIA

Erythroid cells showing central pallor occupying more than one third the size of red cell are termed hypochromic. Peripheral smears with small red cells (microcytes) and hypochromia may be seen in the following:

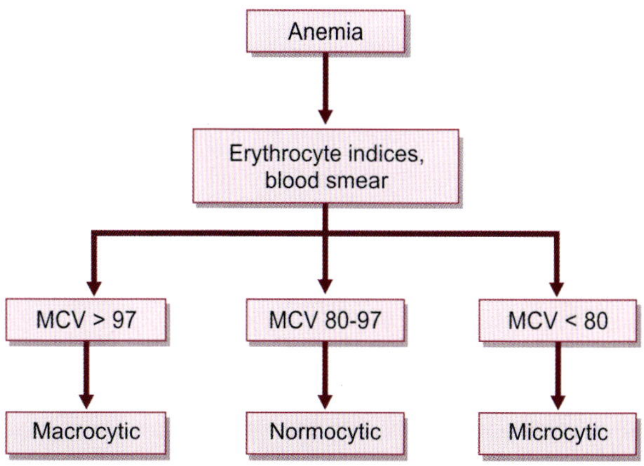

Fig. 1.1: Initial step in the morphologic classification of anemia (microcytic, macrocytic, normocytic anemia)

Iron Deficiency Anemia

- Thalassemia/Hemoglobinopathy
- Sideroblastic anemia
- Anemia of chronic disorder

A good peripheral smear examination in conjunction with hemogram can help diagnose iron deficiency anemia. Presence of microcytic hypochromic red cells (Fig. 1.2) in the absence of target cells, basophilic stippling suggest untreated iron deficiency especially when it is associated with reactive thrombocytosis. Moreover, unlike thalassemia minor, the red cell changes in iron deficiency manifest only when hemoglobin is less than 10 g/dl. Some times elongated pencil cells are also seen in iron deficiency anemia. There may be associated eosinophilia if iron deficiency is secondary to worm infestation.

It may sometimes be difficult to differentiate iron deficiency anemia from anemia of chronic disorder. This may require estimation of bone marrow iron which is assessed on iron stain. Interpretation of bone marrow iron stain is as follows:

- Iron deficiency is the most common cause of anemia worldwide
- Normal (Western) diet provides approximately 15 mg of iron (Fe)/d, of which five to ten percent is absorbed in duodenum and upper jejunum
- Total body iron store is ≈ 4 g. Around 1 mg of iron (Fe)/d is lost in urine, feces, sweat and cells shed from the skin and GIT
- Iron deficiency is more common in the reproductive age since menstrual losses account for ~20 mg Fe/month and in pregnancy an additional 500 to 1000 mg Fe may be lost (transferred from mother to fetus)
- In general, iron metabolism is balanced between absorption of 1 mg/d and loss of 1 mg/d. Pregnancy may also upset the iron balance, since requirements increase to 2 to 5 mg of Fe/d during pregnancy and lactation
- Normal dietary iron cannot supply these requirements, and medicinal iron is needed during pregnancy and lactation. Repeated pregnancy (especially with breastfeeding) may cause iron deficiency if increased requirements are not met with supplemental medicinal iron.

Causes of Iron Deficiency

- *Reproductive system*: Menorrhagia
- *GI tract:* Esophagitis, esophageal varices, hiatus hernia

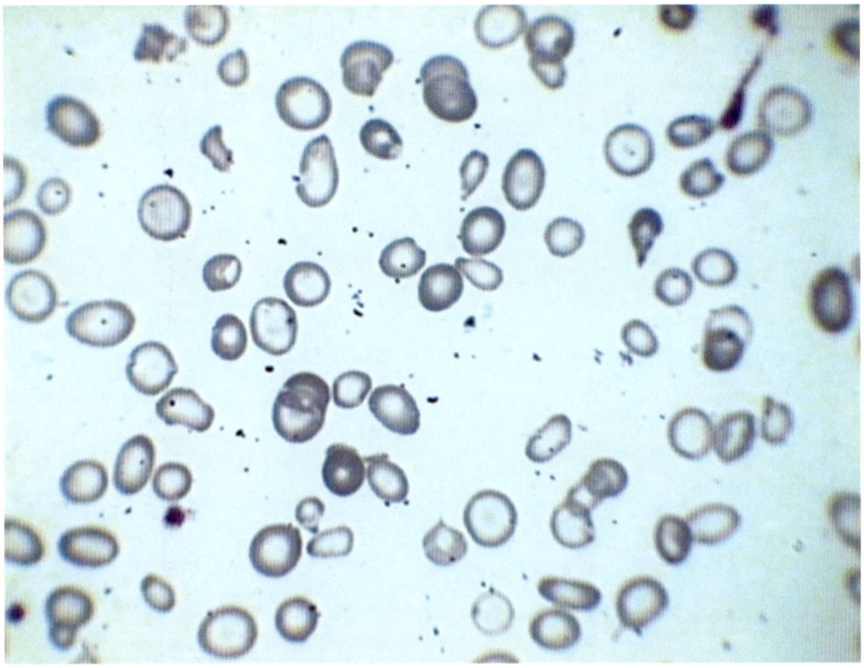

Fig. 1.2: IDA: Microcytic hypochromic

(ulcerated), peptic ulcer, inflammatory bowel disease, hemorrhoids, carcinoma: stomach, colorectal, (rarely angiodysplasia, hereditary hemorrhagic telangiectasia)

- *Malabsorption:* Coeliac disease, atrophic gastritis (*note*: may also result from Fe deficiency), gastrectomy
- *Physiological:* Growth spurts, pregnancy
- *Dietary:* Vegans, elderly
- *Genitourinary system:* Hematuria (uncommon cause)
- *Others:* PNH, frequent venesection, e.g. blood donation

Worldwide Commonest cause is hookworm infestation

Clinical Features

- Symptoms of iron deficiency anemia are those of the anemia itself (easy fatigability, tachycardia, palpitations and tachypnea on exertion).
- Severe deficiency causes skin and mucosal changes, including a smooth tongue, brittle nails and cheilosis. Dysphagia because of the formation of esophageal webs (Plummer–Vinson syndrome) also occurs. In chronic cases, we can see koilonychias (Fig. 1.3).
- Many iron-deficient patients develop pica, craving for specific foods (ice chips, etc.) often not rich in iron.

Treatment

- *Oral iron therapy* should begin with a ferrous iron salt, taken separately from meals in three or four divided doses and supplying a daily total of 150 to 200 mg of elemental iron in adults or 3 mg of iron per kilogram of body weight in children
- Simple ferrous preparations are the best absorbed and least expensive. Ferrous sulfate is the most widely used, either as tablets containing 60 to 70 mg of iron for adults or as a liquid preparation for children
- Administration between meals maximizes absorption
- While the various preparations contain different amounts

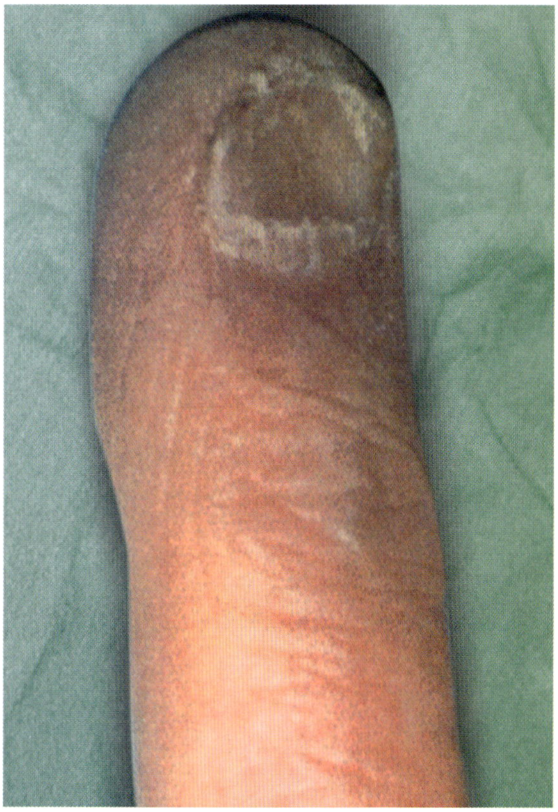

Fig. 1.3: A patient with chronic iron deficiency anemia with koilonychia

of iron, they are generally all absorbed well and are effective in treatment

- An appropriate response is a return of the hematocrit level halfway toward normal within three weeks with full return to baseline after two months
- Iron therapy should continue for 3 to 6 months after restoration of normal hematologic values to replenish iron stores.

Parenteral Iron

- Intravenous iron can be given to patients who are unable to tolerate oral iron, whose needs are relatively acute, or who needs iron on an ongoing basis, usually due to persistent gastrointestinal blood loss
- Parenteral iron use has been rising rapidly in the last several years with the recognition that recombinant erythropoietin therapy induces a large demand for iron
- Total dose of parenteral iron required is calculated by following formula: Body weight (kg) × 2.3 × (15– patient's hemoglobin, g/dl) + 500 or 1000 mg (for stores)
- Iron sucrose (Venofer) or iron dextran prepration are available for intravenous use. Iron sucrose appears to be safer than dextran and no episode of anaphylaxis been reported.

Grading Iron Stains in Bone Marrow Aspirates (Table 1.1)

SIDEROBLASTIC ANEMIA

It is a heterogeneous group of disorders characterized by anemia of varying severity and diagnosed by finding ring sideroblasts in bone marrow aspirate (Fig. 1.4) defined as siderotic granules arranged in a perinuclear collar distribution surrounding one-third or more of the nuclear perimeter.

Iron overload is the common clinical feature and in severe cases may lead to secondary hemosiderosis.

Classification of Sideroblastic Anemia

Hereditary

- X-linked
- Autosomal dominant or recessive

Acquired

- Idiopathic acquired (RARS)
- Associated with previous chemotherapy, irradiation or in "transitional" MDS or MPNs

Drugs

- Alcohol

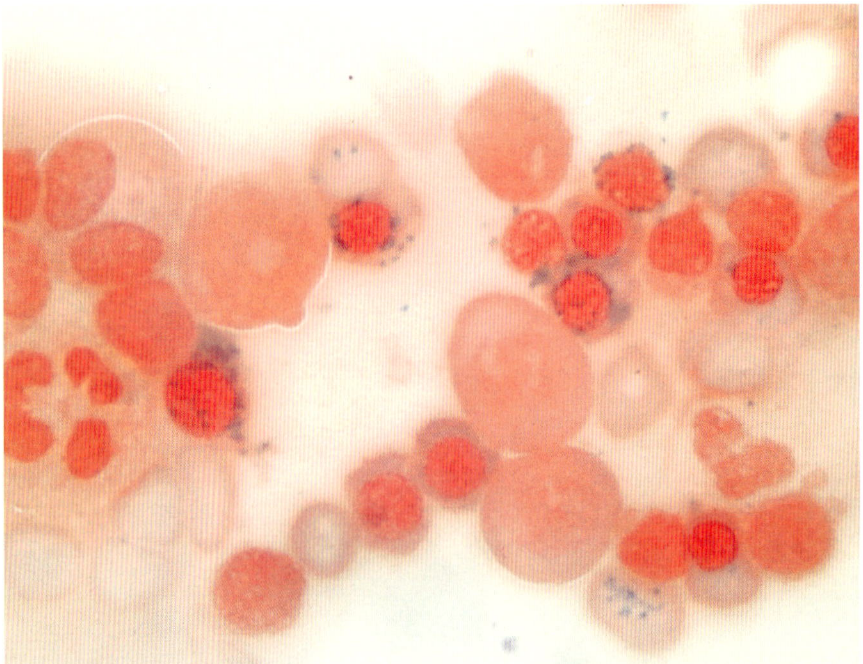

Fig. 1.4: Sideroblastic anemia

Table 1.1: Bone marrow iron positive: Prussian blue stain

Grade	Criteria	Iron content (ug/g)*
0	No iron granules observed	43 ± 23
1+	Small granules in reticulum cells, seen only with oil-immersion lens	130 ± 50
2+	Few small granules visible with low-power lens	223 ± 75
3+	Numerous small granules in all marrow particles	406 ± 131
4+	Large granules in small clumps	762 ± 247
5+	Dense, large clumps of granules	1618 ± 464
6+	Very large deposits, obscuring marrow details.	3681 ± 1400

* Mean ± SD.

- Isoniazid
- Chloramphenicol
- Other drugs

Rare Causes

- Erythropoietic protoporphyria
- Pearson syndrome
- Copper deficiency or zinc overload
- Thiamine responsive megaloblastic anemia
- Hypothermia

MACROCYTIC ANEMIA

This is diagnosed when MCV is greater than 97 fl. MCV >110 highly suggests megaloblastic anemia (MA) whereas < 110 may be seen in aplastic anemia, MDS, liver disease, high reticulocyte count and CDA in addition to megaloblastic anemia. In megaloblastic anemia, peripheral smear may show macrocytes along with fully hemoglobinated macro-ovalocytes, cabot rings, hypersegmented polymorphonuclear cells (1/100 PMN with greater or equal to 6 lobes or 5/100 PMNs with 5 lobes) and rarely circulating megaloblast (Fig. 1.5).

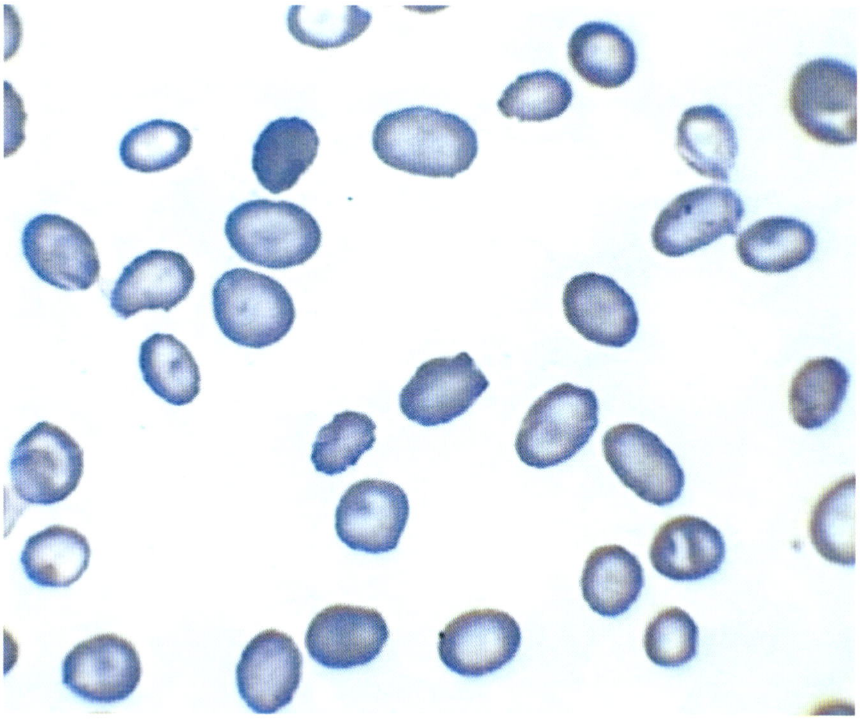

Fig. 1.5: Peripheral smear from a patient with megaloblastic anemia showing macrocytes and macro-ovalocytes (without central pallor)

In cases of doubt, therapeutic response to vitamin B_{12} (1000 mg) and 5 mg folic acid for seven days can be assessed by repeating reticulocyte count which peaks at five to eight days of therapy. Sometimes, macrocytic anemia may be nonmegaloblastic.

B_{12} Deficiency

- The hallmark of symptomatic vitamin B_{12} deficiency is megaloblastic anemia. In advanced cases, the anemia may be severe, with hematocrits as low as 10 to 15 percent and may be accompanied by leukopenia and thrombocytopenia
- Patients are usually pale and may be mildly icteric
- The megaloblastic state also produces changes in mucosal cells, leading to glossitis, as well as other vague gastrointestinal disturbances such as anorexia and diarrhea. Patients can have pigmentation of skins (Fig. 1.6)
- Vitamin B_{12} deficiency also leads to a complex neurologic syndrome. Peripheral nerves are usually affected first and patients complain initially of paresthesias. The posterior columns next become impaired and patients complain of difficulty with balance
- In more advanced cases dementia and other neuropsychiatric changes may precede hematologic changes.

Management of B_{12} Deficiency

- Identify and correct cause if possible
- Vitamin B_{12} replacement, 1 mg of intramuscular cyanocobalamin per day (week 1), 1 mg twice weekly (week 2), 1 mg/week for 4 weeks, and then 1 mg/mo for life.

Folic Acid Deficiency

Symptoms and signs: Similar to those of vitamin B_{12} deficiency with megaloblastic anemia and megaloblastic changes in mucosa. However, usually there are none of the neurologic abnormalities associated with vitamin B_{12} deficiency.

Management

- Folic acid 5 mg/d PO
- Treatment of underlying cause, e.g. in coeliac disease folate levels and absorption normalize once patient established on gluten-free diet.

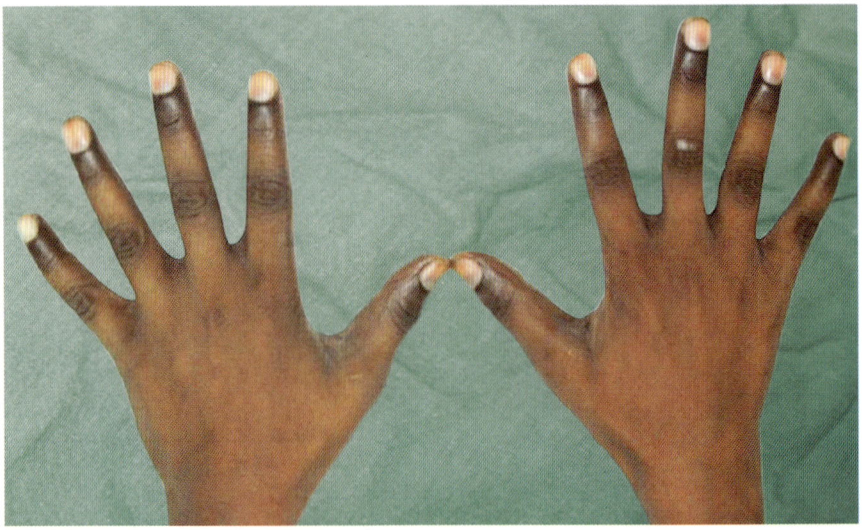

Fig.1.6: Skin pigmentation in megaloblastic anemia

Bone marrow in megaloblastic anemia (Fig. 1.7): This is cellular with erythroid hyperplasia showing nucleocytoplasmic asynchrony. Various stages of erythroblasts are seen with large nuclei, opened out chromatin and relatively hemoglobinized cytoplasm (Fig. 1.7). This is associated with presence of giant myeloid forms and dyserythropoiesis. Although presence of early megaloblastoid changes may be seen in reactive BM, MDS, etc. presence of late megaloblast is generally seen in megaloblastic anemia.

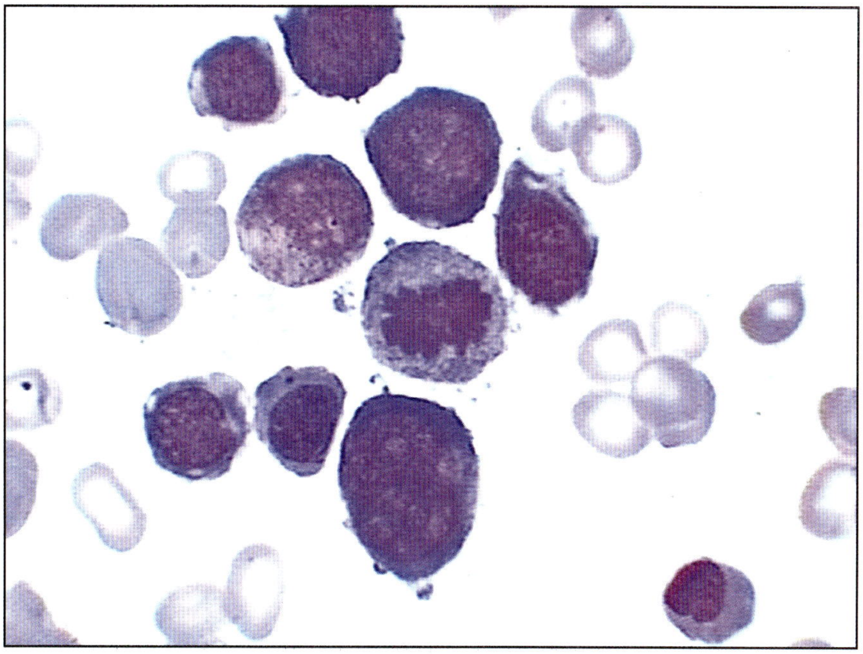

Fig. 1.7: Bone marrow aspirate showing megaloblast with large nucleus with sieve like chromatin and deep blue cytoplasm

DIMORPHIC ANEMIA

At times IDA coexists with megaloblastic anemia. It then shows presence of microcytic as well as macrocytic red cells. Sometimes, red cell morphology due to one deficiency predominates over the other. In such a situation, the other deficiency red cell changes manifest after the first deficiency is treated (Fig. 1.8).

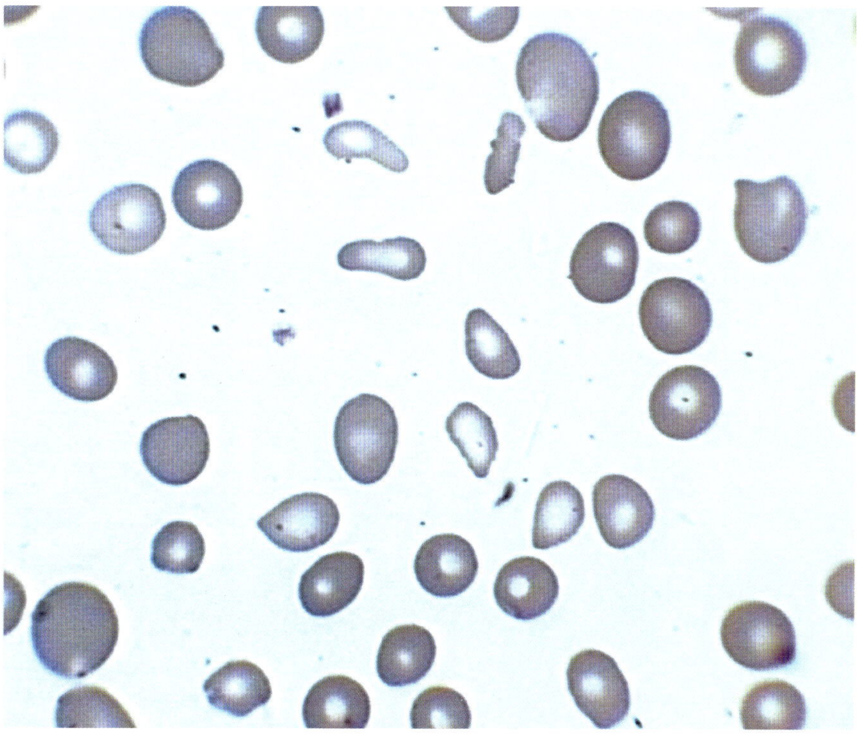

Fig. 1.8: Dimorphic anemia. Presence of microcytic hypochromic, macro-ovalocytes, suggests a combined IDA with megaloblastic anemia

MYELODYSPLASTIC SYNDROME (MDS)

Myelodysplastic syndrome (MDS) is a heterogeneous group of refractory anemias which are clonal stem cell disorders and are characterized by ineffective hematopoiesis, morphologic abnormalities in the bone marrow and the risk of evolution to acute leukemia. The natural history of these disorders is variable and ranges from a chronic to a rapid course towards leukemic progression.

Morphology

Morphologic dysplasia in any cell-line showing at least in > 10% cells, is considered significant.

- Erythroid series dysplastic features:
  - Macrocyte, macro-ovalocyte, elliptocytes, tear drop cells, Howell-Jolly bodies
  - Basophilic stippling
  - Dimorphic red cells
  - Megaloblastosis, nuclear budding, karyorrhexis, vacuolization, nuclear bridging (Figs 1.9 and 1.10)
  - Ringed sideroblasts
  - PAS +ve erythroblasts

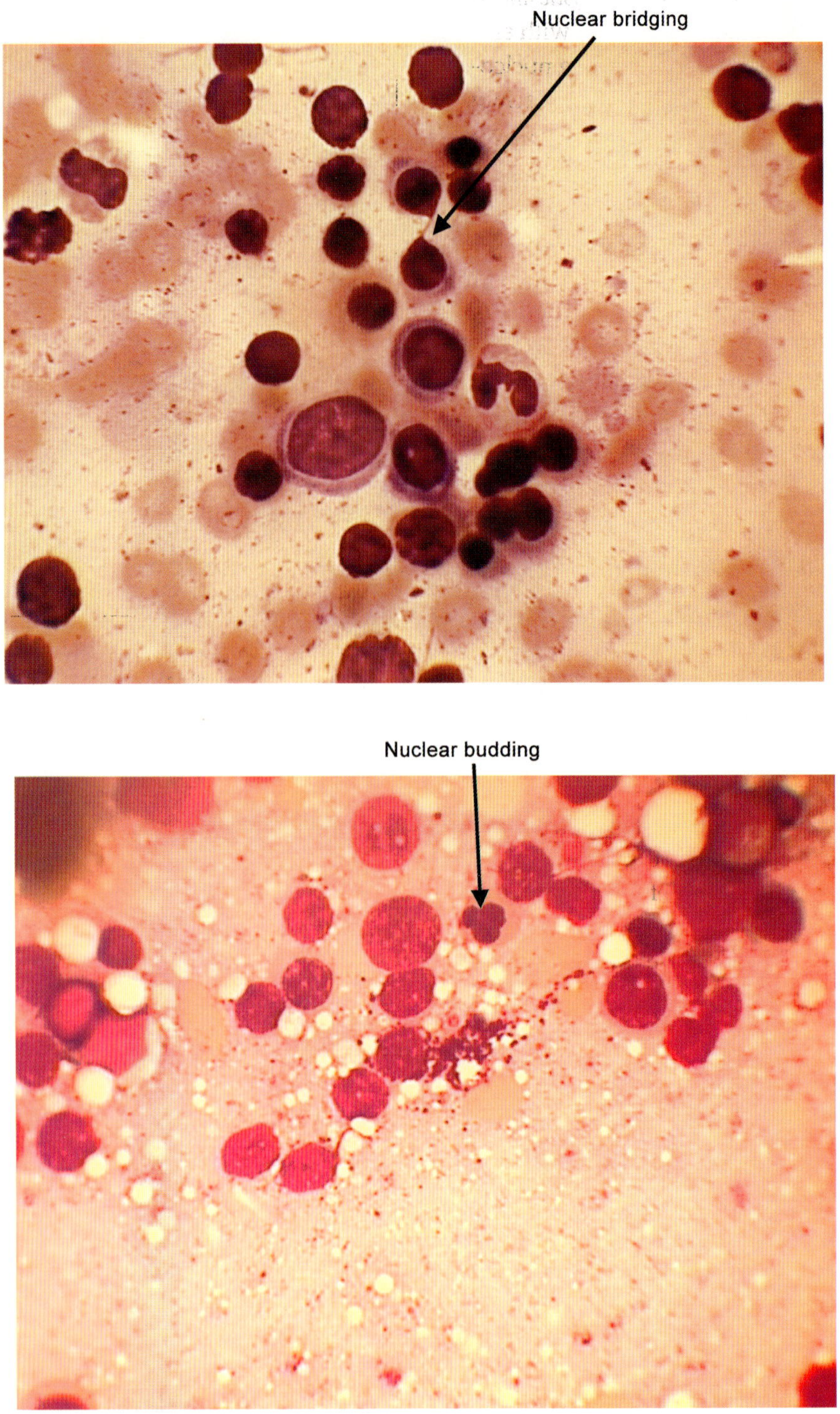

Fig. 1.9: Bone marrow aspirate showing dyserythropoiesis in the forms of nuclear bridging and budding

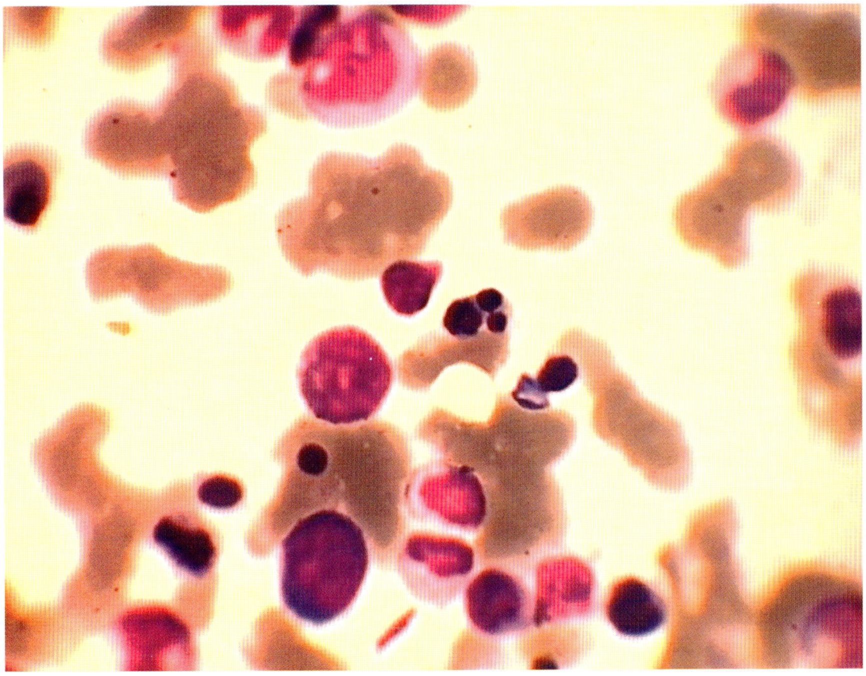

Fig. 1.10: Dyserythropoiesis

- Granulocyte series dysplastic features
  - Poor or abnormal granulation
  - Decreased LAP score and peroxidase
  - Pseudo-Pelger-Huet anomaly (which represents apoptotic neutrophils) (Fig. 1.11)

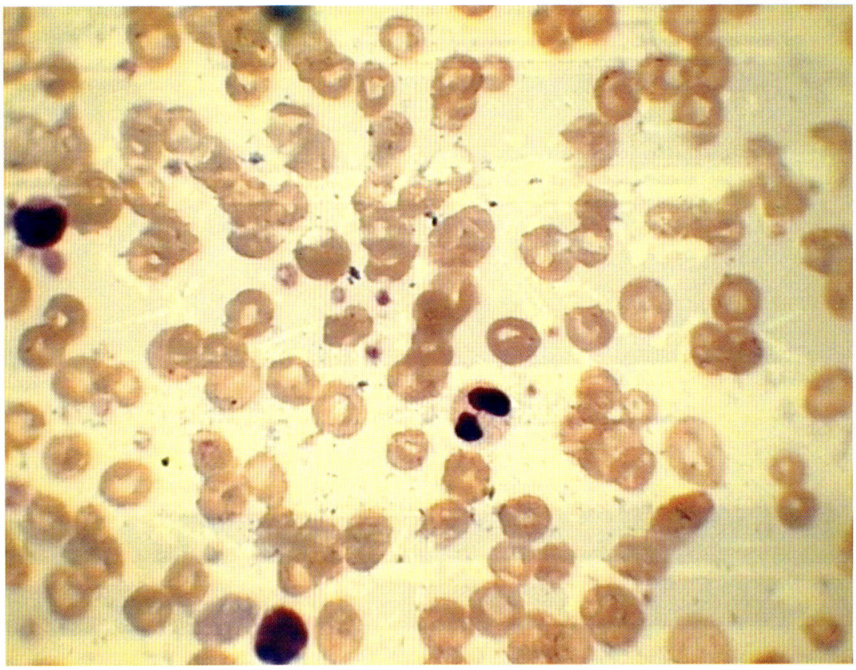

Fig.1.11: Peripheral smear showing dysmyelopoiesis in neutrophil in the pseudo-Pelger-Huet anomaly (2 lobes)

- Hypersegmentation of neutrophils (Figs 1.12 and 1.13A and B)
- Pseudo-Chediak-Higashi granules
- Nucleolated myelocytes (Figs 1.13A and B)

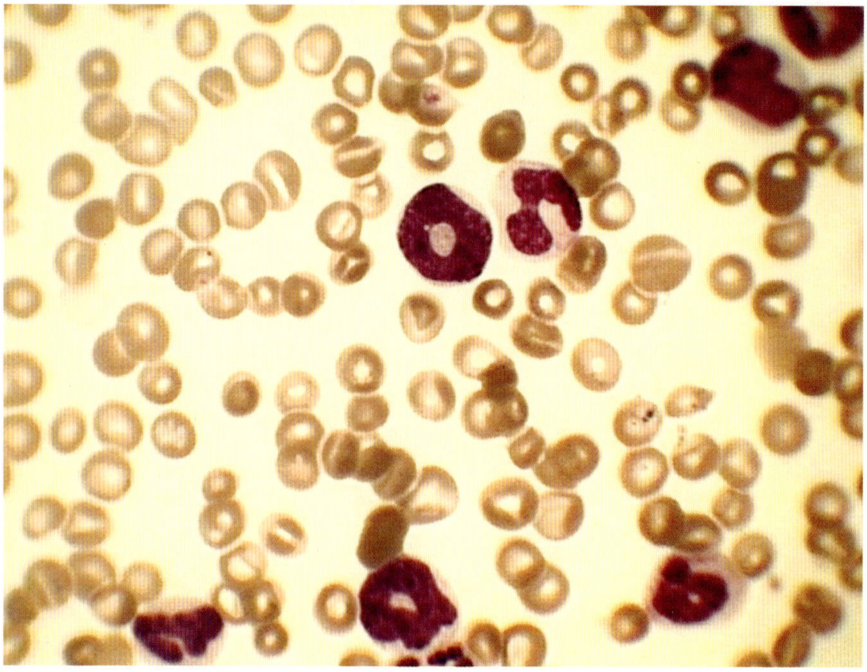

Fig. 1.12: Peripheral smear showing dysmyelopoiesis in the form of ring neutrophil

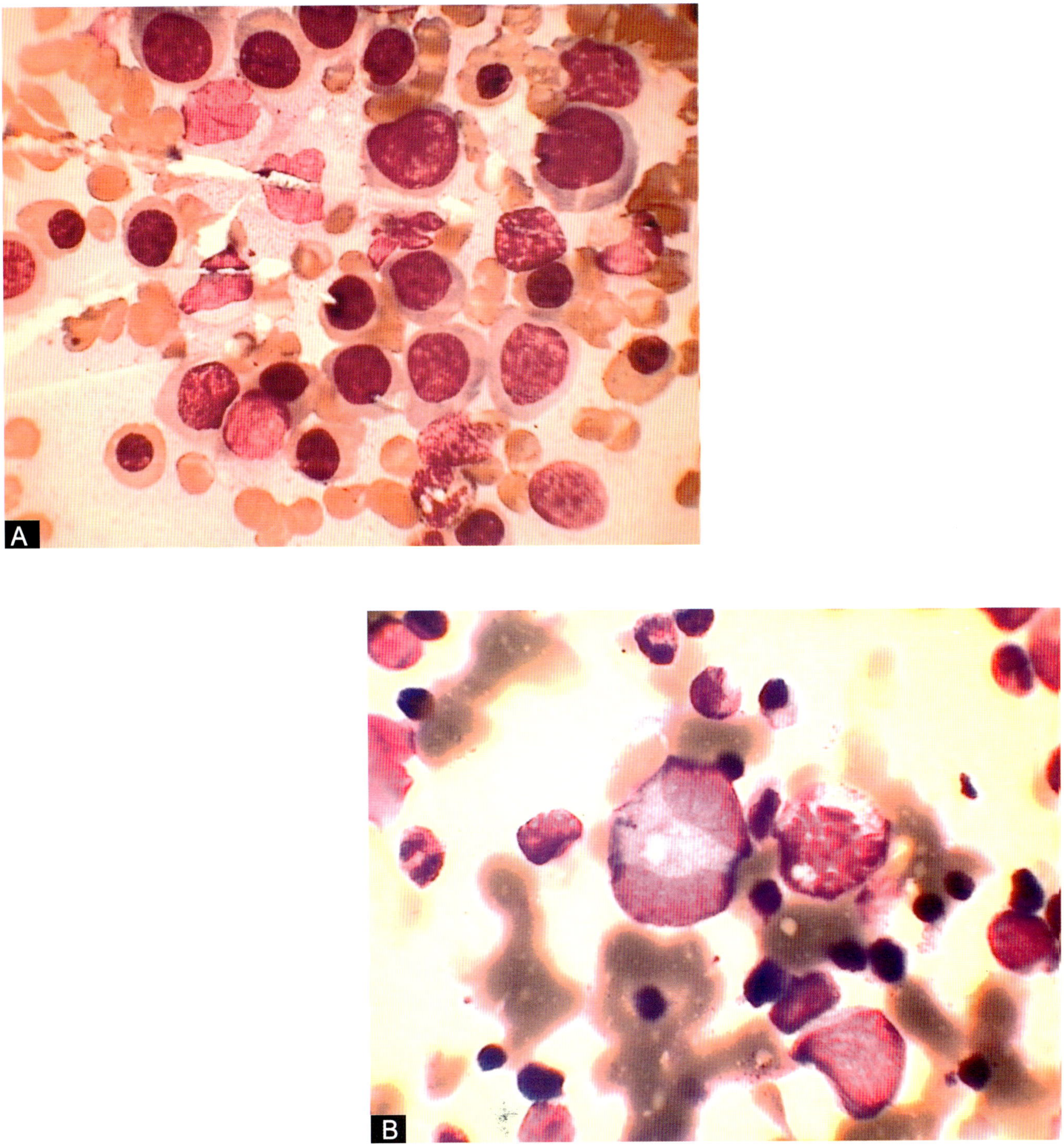

Figs 1.13A and B: Bone marrow showing dysmyelopoiesis in form of nucleolated myelocyte

- Bone marrow show dysmyelopoiesis wiht increased blasts (Figs 1.14 and 1.15)

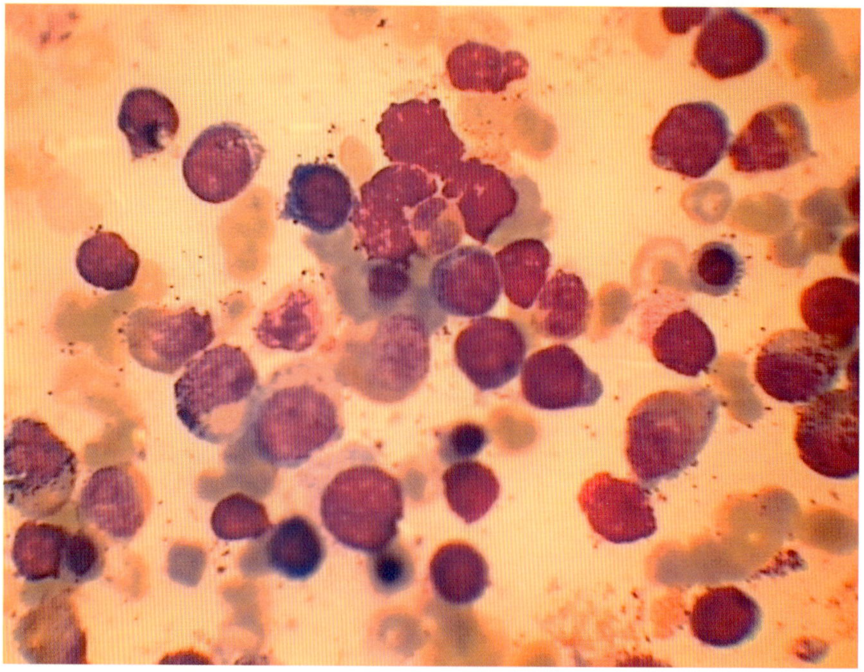

Fig. 1.14: Bone marrow from refractory anemia with excess blast (RAEB-1) showing dysmyelopoiesis with blasts with between 5% and 10%

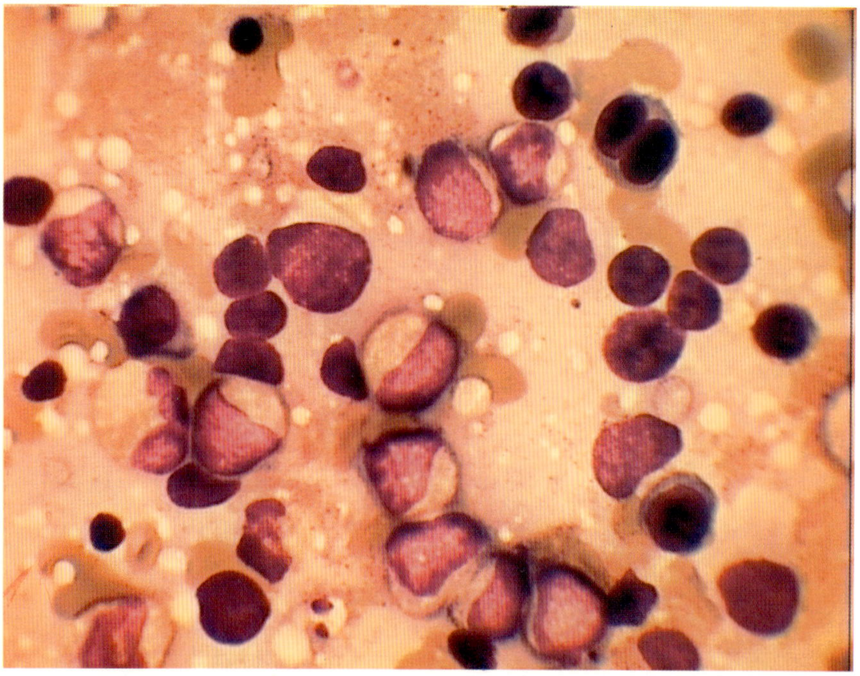

Fig. 1.15: Bone marrow from refractory anemia with excess blast in transfomation (RAEB-2) showing; dysmyelopoiesis with blasts between 10% and 20%

- Platelets/megakaryocytes dysplastic features (Fig. 1.16)
  - Anisocytosis with presence of giant and bizarre platelets
  - Agranular platelets
  - Presence of hypolobulated micromegakaryocytes (Fig. 1.17)

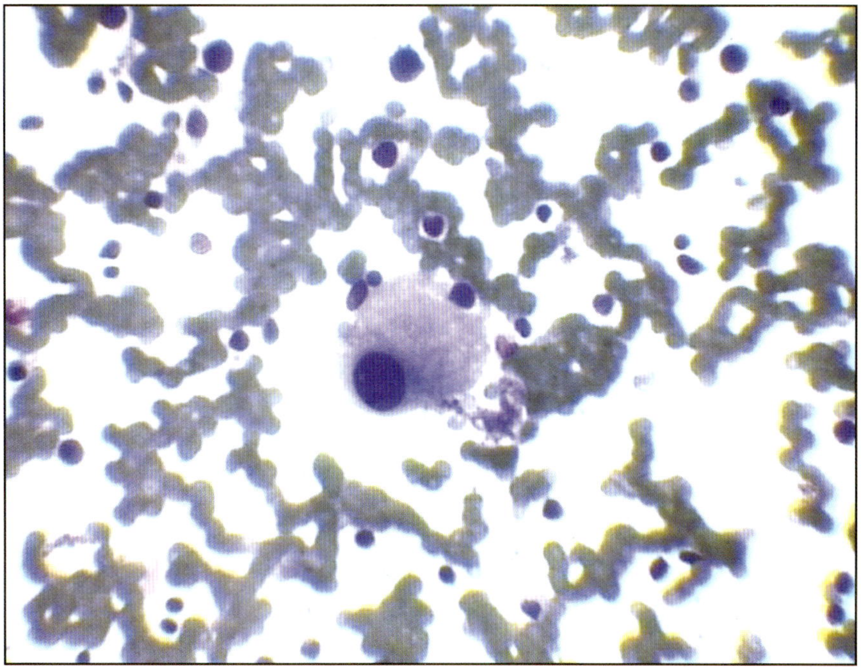

Fig. 1.16: Bone marrow from a patient with 5q-syndrome showing dysplastic megakaryocytes

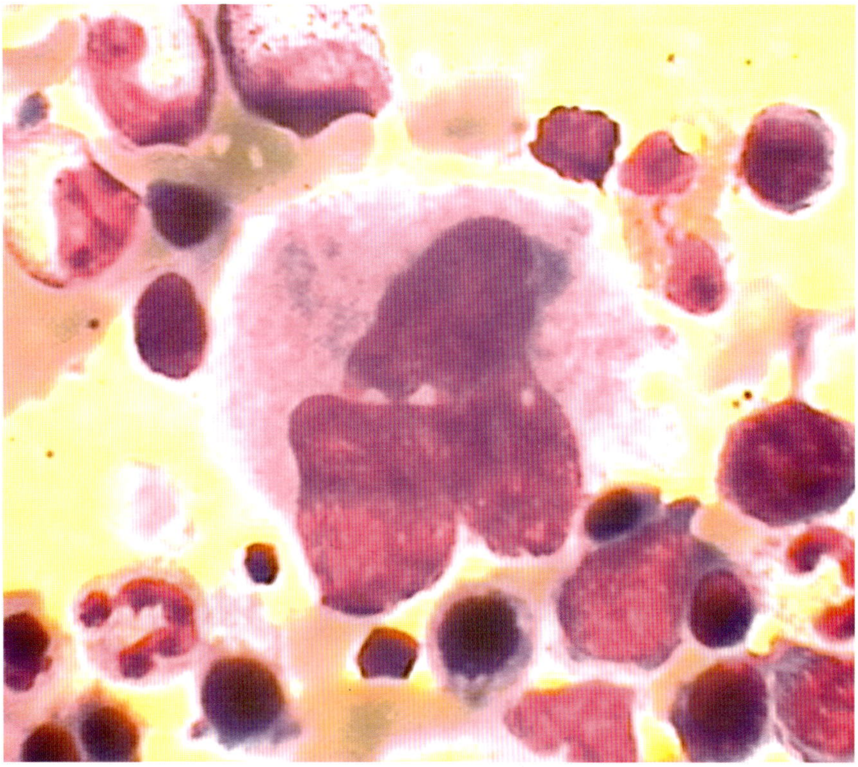

Fig. 1.17: Dysmegakaryopoiesis showing micromegakaryocyte with odd number of lobes in the nucleus

- Megakaryocytes with a large, single lobed nucleus or having odd number of lobes.
- Hypogranular megakaryocytes.
- Megakaryocytes with widely separated nuclei (Figs 1.18A and B)

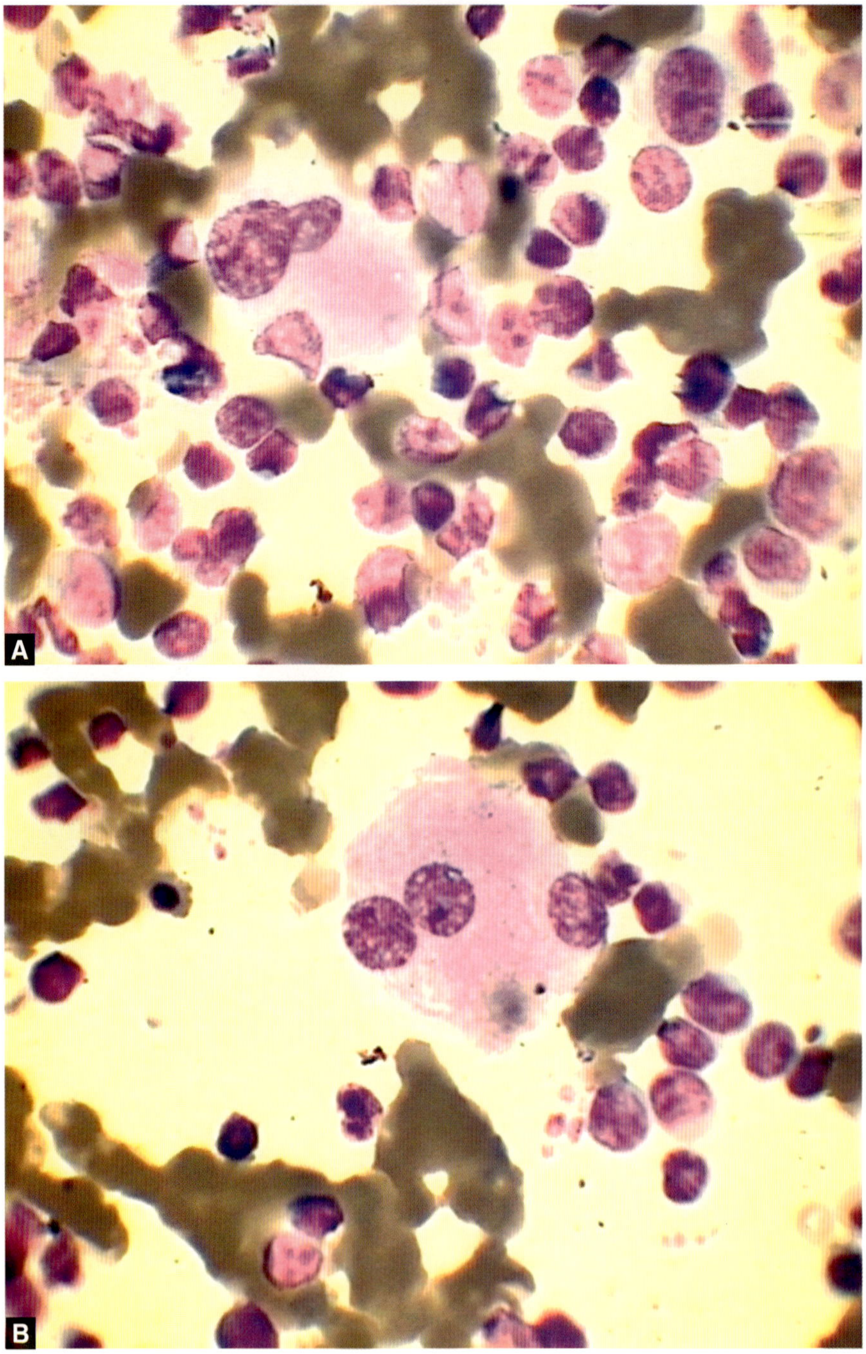

Figs 1.18A and B: Dysmegakaryopoiesis with separated micromegakaryocyte lobes

- 5q syndrome
  - This is a type of MDS characterised by thrombocytosis and macrocytosis in peripheral smear (Fig. 1.19)
  - Bone marrow shows dysplastic megakaryocytes (Fig. 1.16)
  - Cytogenetics show characteristic deletion of long arm of chromosome 5
  - It is important to identify as the patient responds to lenalidomide

NORMOCYTIC NORMOCHROMIC ANEMIA

This anemia includes aplastic anemia hemolytic anemia (Given in other chapters).

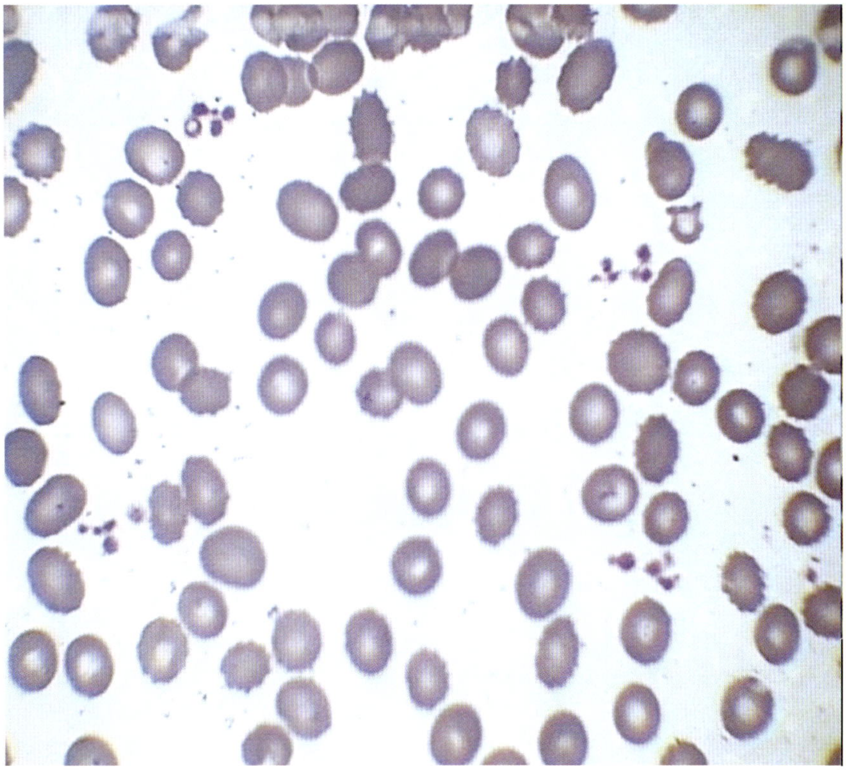

Fig. 1.19: Peripheral smear from a patient with 5q-syndrome showing thrombocytosis

CHAPTER 2

Bone Marrow Failure Syndromes

CHAPTER OVERVIEW

- Aplastic anemia
- Differential diagnosis of pancytopenia
- Fanconi's anemia
- Paroxysmal nocturnal hemoglobinuria (PNH)
- Pure red cell aplasia (PRCA)

APLASTIC ANEMIA

This is a stem cell disorder where the peripheral smear shows pancytopenia and the bone biopsy shows less than 30 percent cellularity. Depending on the alterations in the various parameters, aplastic anemia can be subclassified as severe, very severe and non-severe.

Aplastic Anemia with Patchy Cellularity

Sometimes there is patchy cellularity in bone marrow biopsy but the overall cellularity should be less than 25 percent for a diagnosis of aplastic anemia (Figs 2.1 and 2.2).

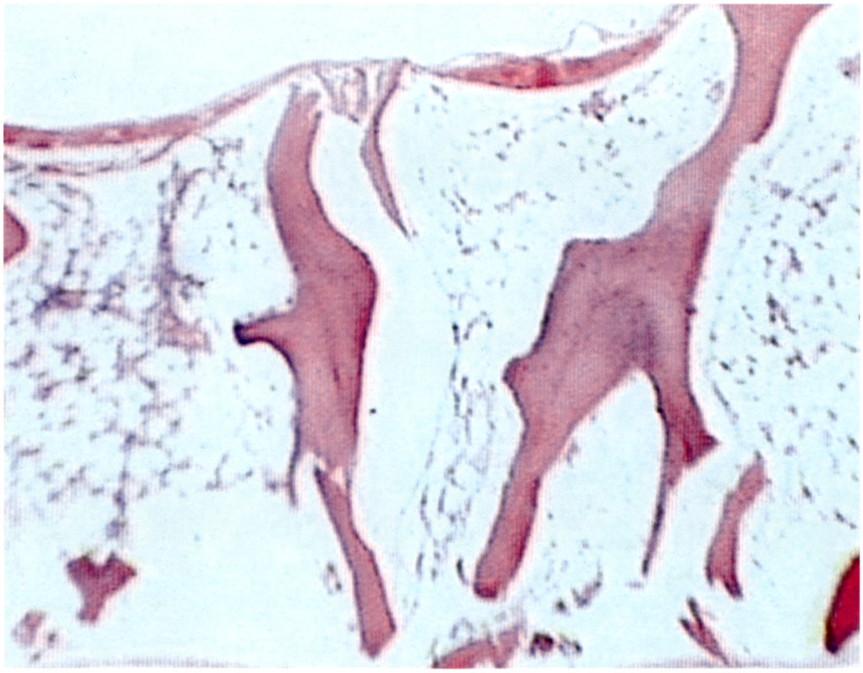

Fig. 2.1: Bone marrow biopsy from aplastic anemia showing < 5% cellularity

Criteria for Aplastic Anemia

Severity of Aplastic Anemia (AA)

Severe

- Bone marrow cellularity <25 percent or 25 to 50 percent with <30 percent residual hematopoietic cells.*
- Two out of three of the following:
  - Neutrophils $<0.5 \times 10^9/l$
  - Platelet $<20 \times 10^9/l$
  - Reticulocytes $<20 \times 10^9/l$

Very Severe

As for severe AA but neutrophils, $0.2 \times 10^9/l$ (Bacigalupo et al. 1988).

Non-severe

- Patients not fulfilling the criteria for severe or very severe aplastic anemia.
- Cellularity should be determined by comparison with normal controls (Tuzuner and Bennet. 1994).

Clinical Features

- Reflects the pancytopenia. Bleeding from mucosal sites common region with purpura (Fig. 2.3)

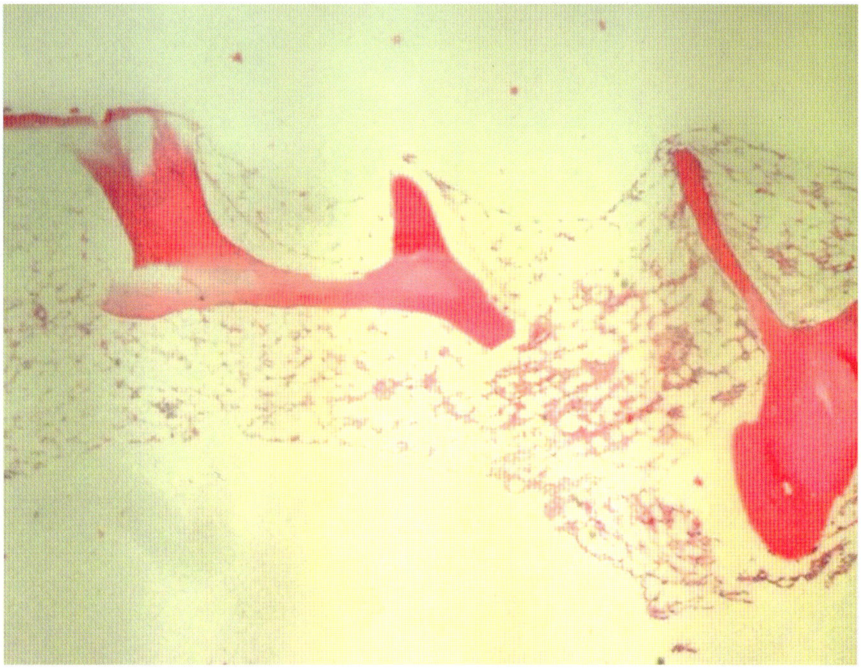

Fig. 2.2: Bone marrow biopsy showing patchy cellularity (overall cellularity : 5-10%)

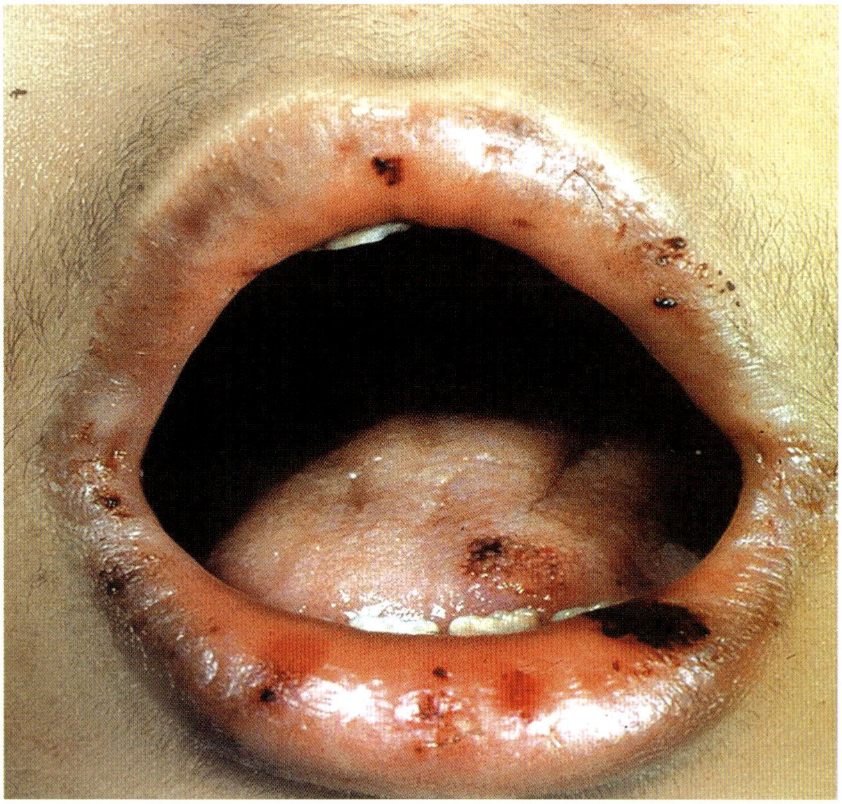

Fig. 2.3: A patient with aplastic anemia with wet-purpura

* Hematopoietic cells include myeloid, erythroid and megakarocytic components

and ecchymoses (Fig. 2.4). Infections, particularly upper and lower respiratory tracts, skin, mouth and perianal. Bacterial (Fig. 2.5) and fungal infections

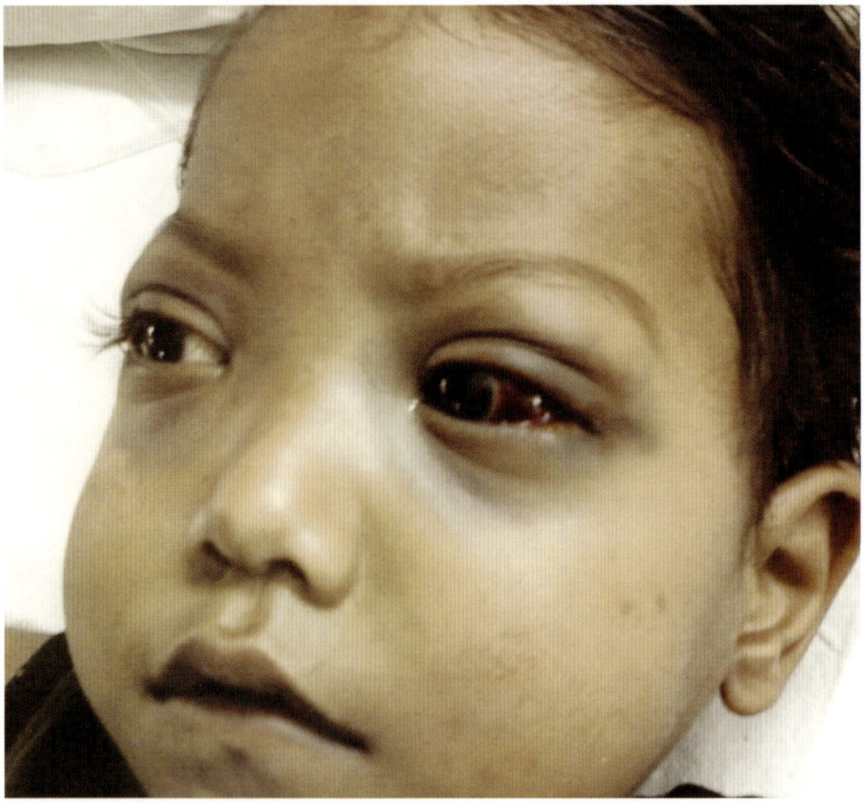

Fig. 2.4: A patient of aplastic anemia with periorbital ecchymosis

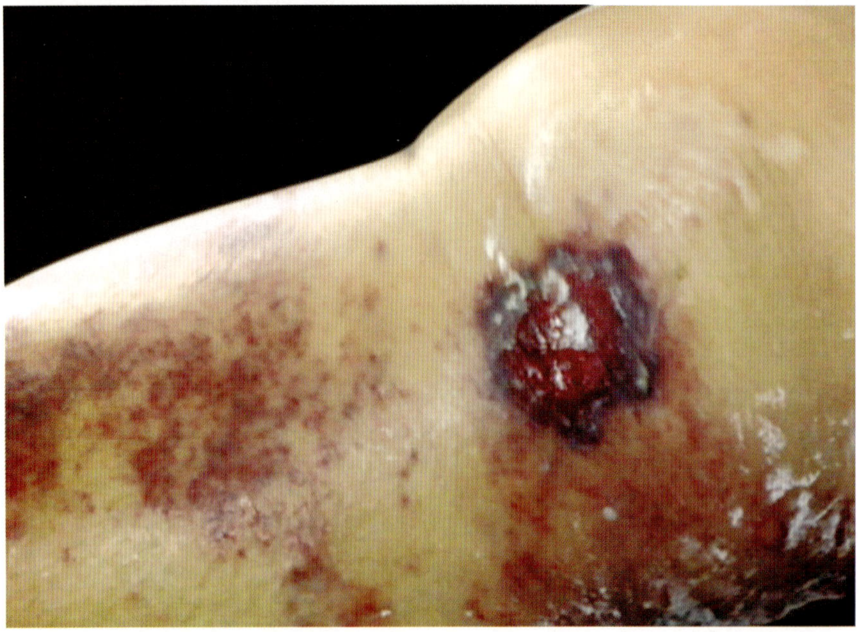

Fig. 2.5: Skin lesions in a patient of aplastic anemia with *pseudomonas septicemia*

common (Figs 2.6 and 2.7). Anemic symptoms usually less severe due to chronic onset

- Physical examination may reveal signs of pallor, purpura and petechiae. Presence of hepatosplenomegaly, lymphadenopathy or bone tenderness should lead to questioning of the diagnosis.

DIFFERENTIAL DIAGNOSIS OF PANCYTOPENIA

Pancytopenia with Hypocellular Bone Marrow

- Acquired aplastic anemia
- Inherited aplastic anemia (Fanconi's anemia and others)
- Some myelodysplasia syndromes
- Rare aleukemic leukemia (acute myelogenous leukemia)
- Some acute lymphoblastic leukemias
- Some lymphomas of bone marrow.

Pancytopenia with Cellular Bone Marrow

Primary Bone Marrow Diseases

- Myelodysplasia syndromes
- Paroxysmal nocturnal hemoglobinuria
- Myelofibrosis
- Some aleukemic leukemias
- Myelophthisis
- Bone marrow lymphoma
- Hairy cell leukemia.

Secondary to Systemic Diseases

- Systemic lupus erythematosus, Sjögren's syndrome
- Hypersplenism
- Vitamin B_{12}, folate deficiency (familial defect)

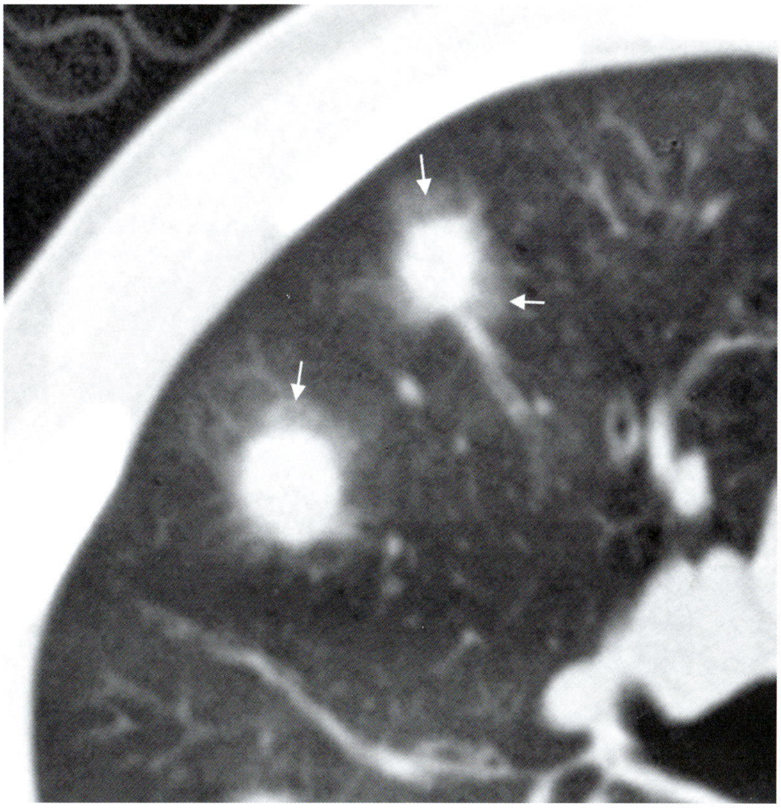

Fig. 2.6: Chest X-ray showing "halo sign" classical of invasive fungal infections

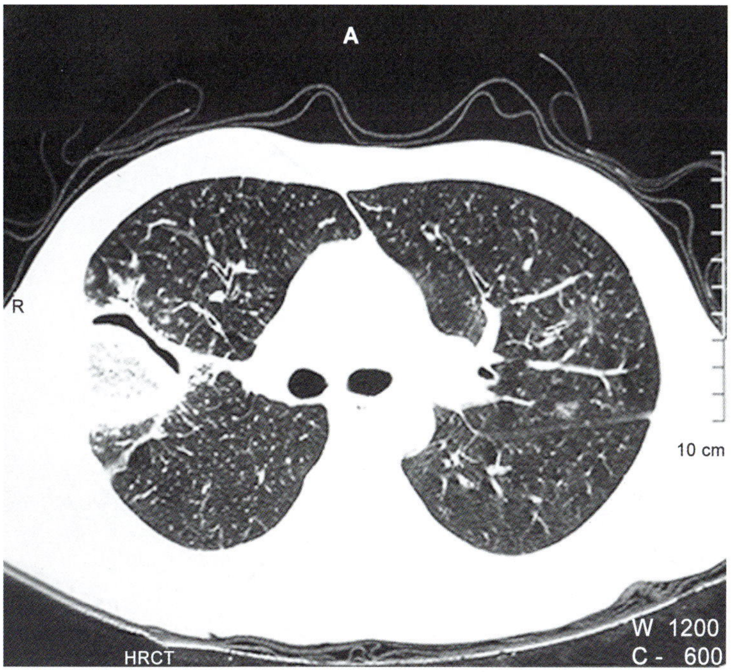

Fig. 2.7: CT scan of chest showing "crescent sign" in right-sided lung field suggesting invasive fungal infections

- Overwhelming infection
- Alcohol
- Brucellosis
- Ehrlichiosis
- Sarcoidosis
- Tuberculosis and atypical mycobacteria.

Complications

- Progression to more severe disease
- Evolutions to PNH—occur in 7 percent
- Transformations to acute leukemia occur in 5 to 10 percent.

Treatment

- Mild cases need careful observation only. More severe will need supportive treatment with red cell and platelet transfusions and antibiotics as needed. Blood products should preferably be leukodepleted to reduce risk of sensitization
- Specific treatment options are between allogeneic transplant and immunosuppression
- Sibling allogeneic transplant is the treatment of choice for those <40 years, if a HLA match sibling is available
- Patients not eligible for transplantation should be treated with combined immunosuppressive therapy with antithyrocyte globulin (ATG/ALG) and cyclosporin. Response rate (60–80%), may take three months. Refractory or relapsing patients may respond to a second course
- Cyclosporin alone has a response rate of 30 to 50 percent
- Androgens or danazol may be useful in some mild cases.

FANCONI'S ANEMIA

- Fanconi's anemia (FA) is a clinically heterogeneous disorder usually presenting in childhood with the common feature being slowly progressive marrow failure affecting all three cell lines (RBC, WBC and megakaryocytes) and eventual marrow aplasia
- FA affects all cells of the body. The cellular phenotype is characterized by increased chromosomal breakage, hypersensitivity to DNA crosslinking agents such as diepoxybutane (DEB) and mitomycin C (MMC), hypersensitivity to oxygen, increased apoptosis and accelerated telomere shortening (Fig. 2.8)

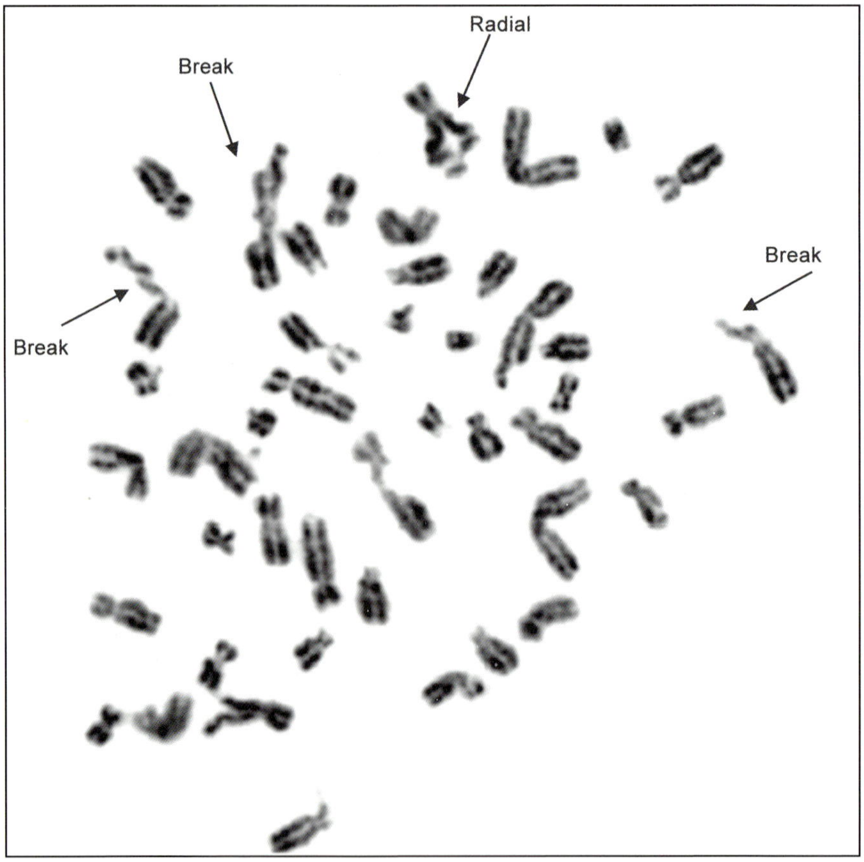

Fig. 2.8: Stress cytogenetics showing breaks suggestive of Fanconi's anemia

- The increased chromosomal fragility is characteristic and used as a diagnostic test
- Apart from progressive marrow failure, 70 percent of FA patients show somatic abnormalities, chiefly involving the skeleton (Fig. 2.9)
- Ninety percent develop marrow failure and survivors show an increased risk of developing leukemia, chiefly AML. Rarely, FA can present as AML. There is also an increased risk of liver tumors and squamous cell carcinomas
- Isolated thrombocytopenia may be first manifestation, lasting two to three years before other cytopenias occur. Ten percent present in adolescence or adult life, four present in early infancy (<1 year).
- Disorders of skin pigmentation common (60%)—Café-au-lait spots (Fig. 2.10), hypo- and hyperpigmentation (Fig. 2.10).
- Short stature in 60 percent, microcephaly, delayed development in >20 percent, skeletal defects common (>50 percent in the upper limb especially absent thumbs, scoliosis, radial hypoplasia) and genitourinary (underdeveloped gonads, horseshoe kidneys)
- Characteristic facies described—elfin-like, with tapering jaw line.

Treatment

- BMT is potentially curative, but FA patients are hypersensitive to conditioning agents cyclophosphamide and radiation. Using lower doses of conditioning, matched sibling grafts give 70 percent actuarial survival

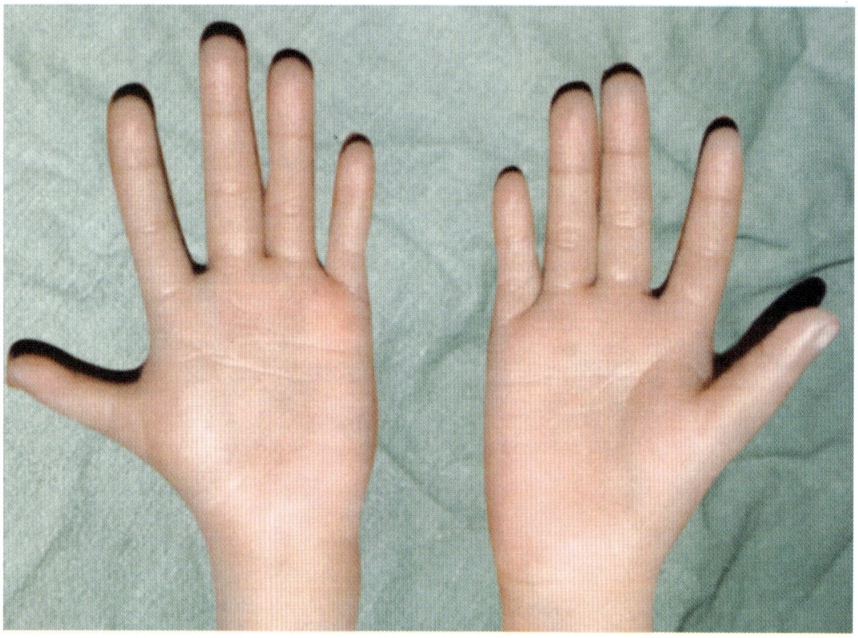

Fig. 2.9: Abnormal thumb of right hand in a patient of Fanconi's anemia

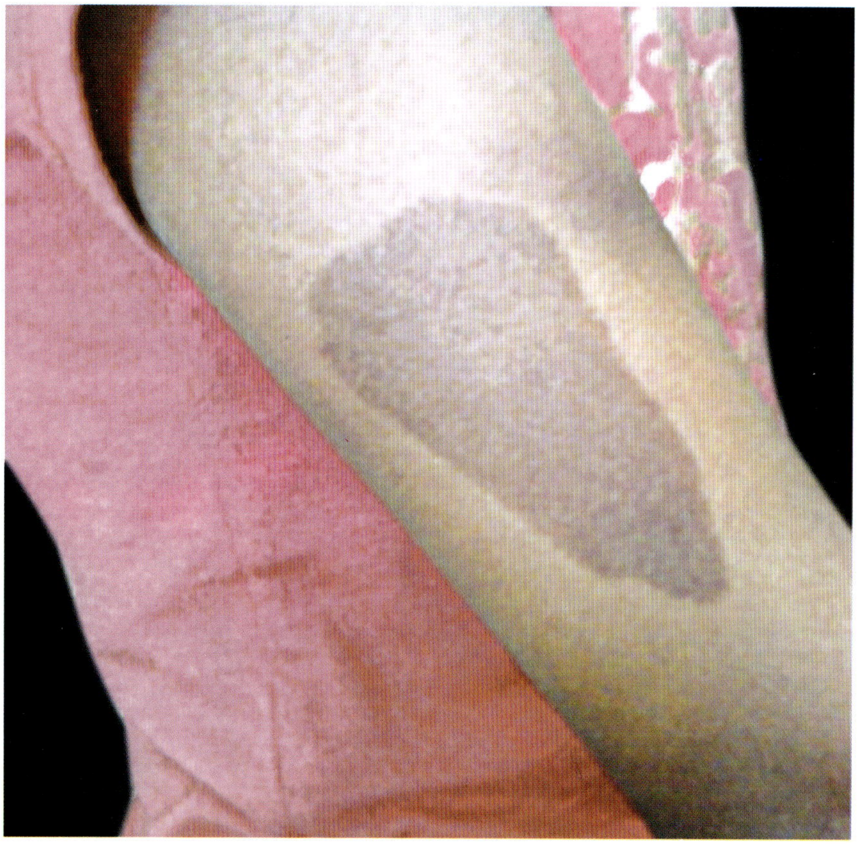

Fig. 2.10: Café-au-lait spot in a patient of Fanconi's anemia

at two years; Early survivors showed four times risk of tumors, especially head and neck

- Androgens (oxymethalone 2–5 mg/kg/d) can be tried in those are not eligible for BMT.

Outcome

- Median survival of conventional treatment responders who do not undergo BMT is ~25 years. Non-responders have a median survival of ~12 years
- Death most commonly due to marrow failure, but 10 to 20 percent will develop MDS or AML after a median period of observation of 13 years.

PAROXYSMAL NOCTURNAL HEMOGLOBINURIA (PNH)

Ten percent of aplastic anemia cases may be associated with PNH. This is diagnosed as a refractory anemia which shows absence of CD55 and CD59 (Fig. 2.11).

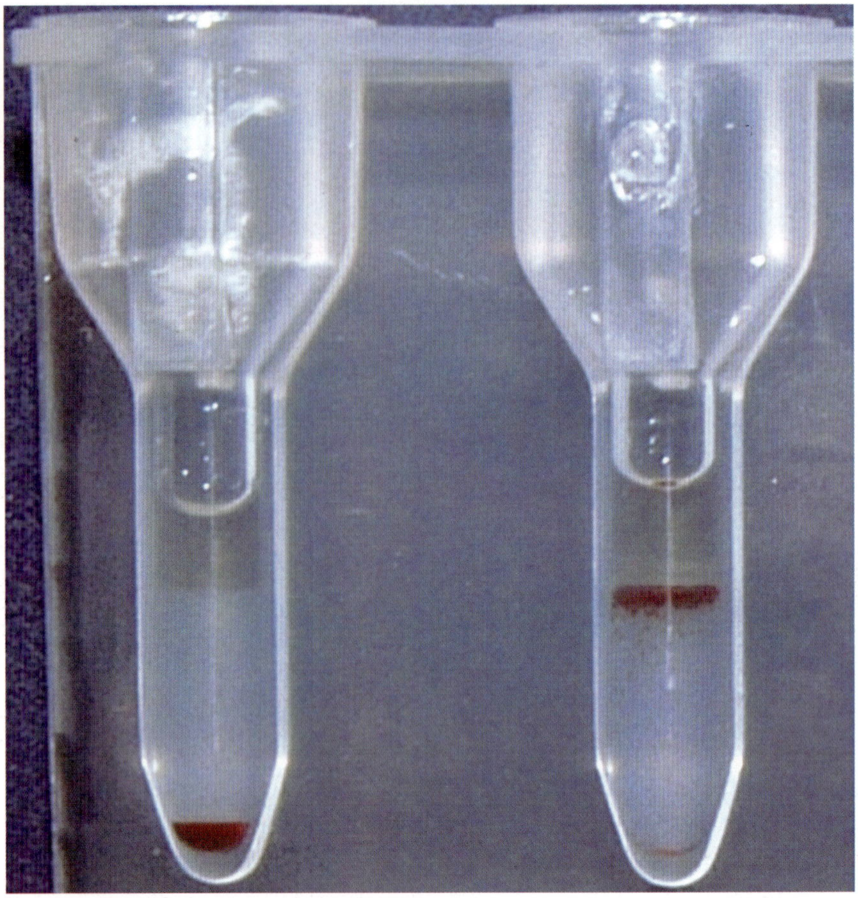

Fig. 2.11: Gel card test of PNH showing absence of CD55/59 on red cells

PURE RED CELL APLASIA (PRCA)

This is an inherited or acquired condition where there is selective paucity of erythroid precursors (Figs 2.12 and 2.13).

It is diagnosed when the percent of

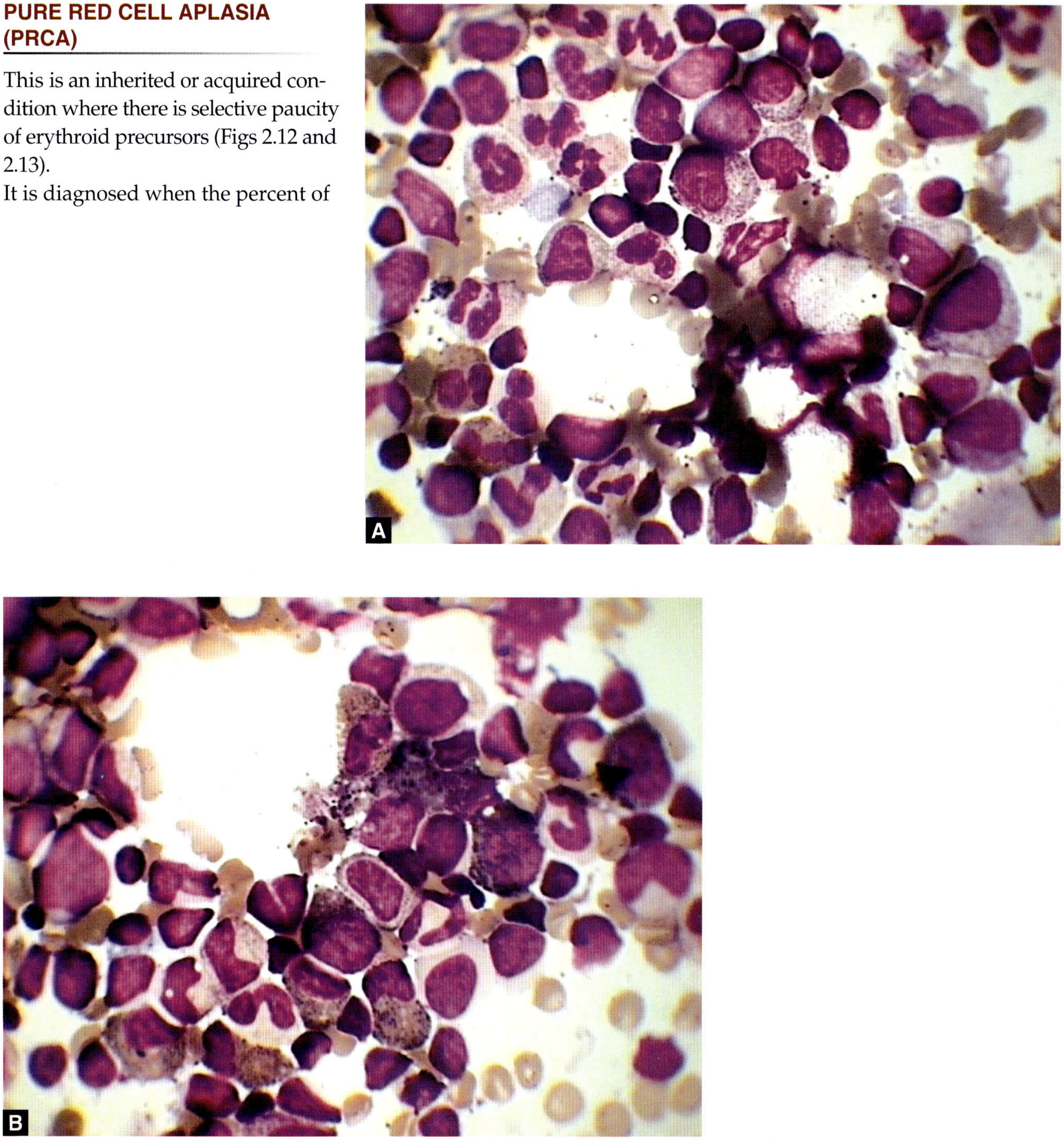

Figs 2.12A and B: Bone marrow aspirate from a case of pure red cell aplasia showing normal myeloid precursors with marked paucity of erythroid precursors

red cell precursors is less than 5% of all cells on bone marrow aspirate and biopsy with preservation of myeloid and megakaryocytic precursors (Figs 2.13A and B). The erythroid precursors present mainly

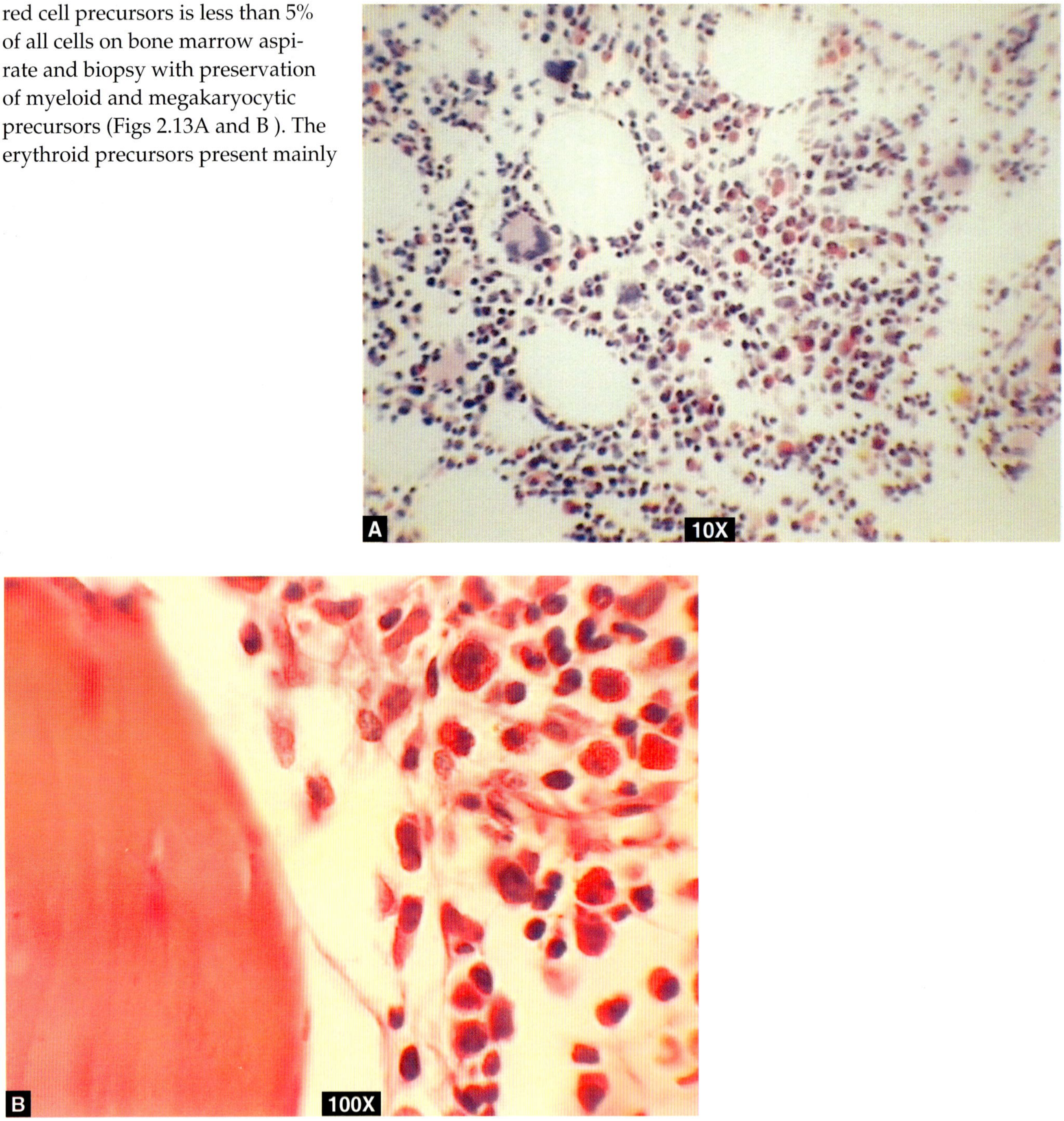

Figs 2.13A and B: Bone biopsy from a case of PRCA showing normal myeloid and megakaryocyte precursors with paucity of erythroid precursors

show early megaloblastoid features. It is important to differentiate this from myeloid hyperplasia due to reaction to infections. Causes of pure red cell aplasia include infections like parvovirus B19. Parvovirus infection in the bone marrow shows presence of early megaloblastoid erythroid precursors with presence of nuclear inclusions and vacuoles in light blue cytoplasm (Fig. 2.14).

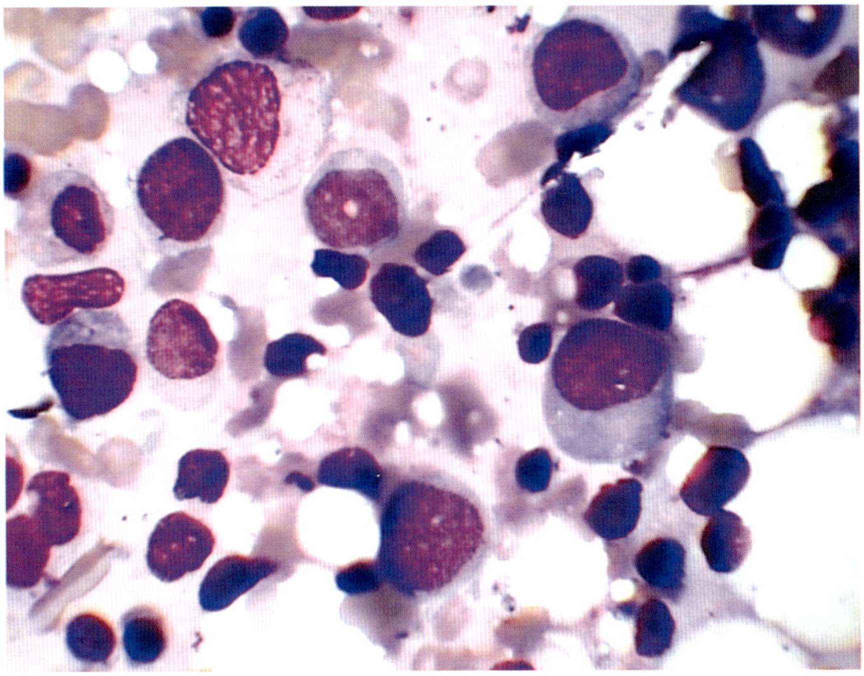

Fig. 2.14: Bone marrow aspirate from a case of parvovirus infection showing erythroid cells with large nucleus, pale blue cytoplasm and intranuclear inclusions

CHAPTER 3

Hemolytic Anemias

CHAPTER OVERVIEW

- Peripheral blood examination
- Diagnosis of Hemoglobinopathies
- Common high perfomance liquid chromatography (HPLC) patterns
- Congenital dyserythropoietic anemia (CDA)
- Thalassemia
- Hereditary spherocytosis

Hemolytic anemias are a heterogeneous group of diseases. They are characterized by reduction in RBC life-span due to increased RBC destruction and failure of compensatory marrow response. They usually present with anemia, icterus (due to unconjugated hyperbilirubinemia), splenomegaly and features of underlying disease (Table 3.1).

Table 3.1: Classification

Intrinsic	
Membrane defects	Hereditary spherocytosis, hereditary elliptocytosis, paroxysmal nocturnal hemoglobinuria
Enzyme defects	Pyruvate kinase deficiency, severe hypophosphatemia, glucose-6-phosphate dehydrogenase deficiency, methemoglobinemia
Hemoglobinopathies	Sickle cell syndromes, unstable hemoglobins, methemoglobinemia
Extrinsic	
Immune	Autoimmune, lymphoproliferative disease, drug toxicity
Microangiopathic	Thrombotic thrombocytopenic purpura, hemolytic-uremic syndrome, disseminated intravascular coagulation, valve hemolysis, metastatic adenocarcinoma, vasculitis
Infection	*Plasmodium, Clostridium, Borrelia*
Others	Hypersplenism, Burns

PERIPHERAL BLOOD EXAMINATION

Peripheral smear examination is of paramount importance in their diagnosis. In many of them diagnosis comes from information of patients family history, clinical presentation and hemogram with peripheral blood smear examination. Bone marrow biopsy is not needed and is only indicated if there is suspicion of aplastic or megaloblastic crisis.

Hemolytic anemia is characterized by presence of polychromasia, red cell fragments, basophilic stippling, nucleated RBC, some time leukoerythroblastosis in peripheral blood and reticulocytosis on supravital staining with methylene blue (Fig. 3.1). The following features in red cell morphology aid in underlying diagnosis:

a. *Spherocytosis:* Peripheral smear shows normocytic normochromic red cells with presence of microspherocytes, small red cells without central pallor (Fig 3.2). These may be seen in the following:
   - Hereditary spherocytosis
   - Autoimmune hemolytic anemia

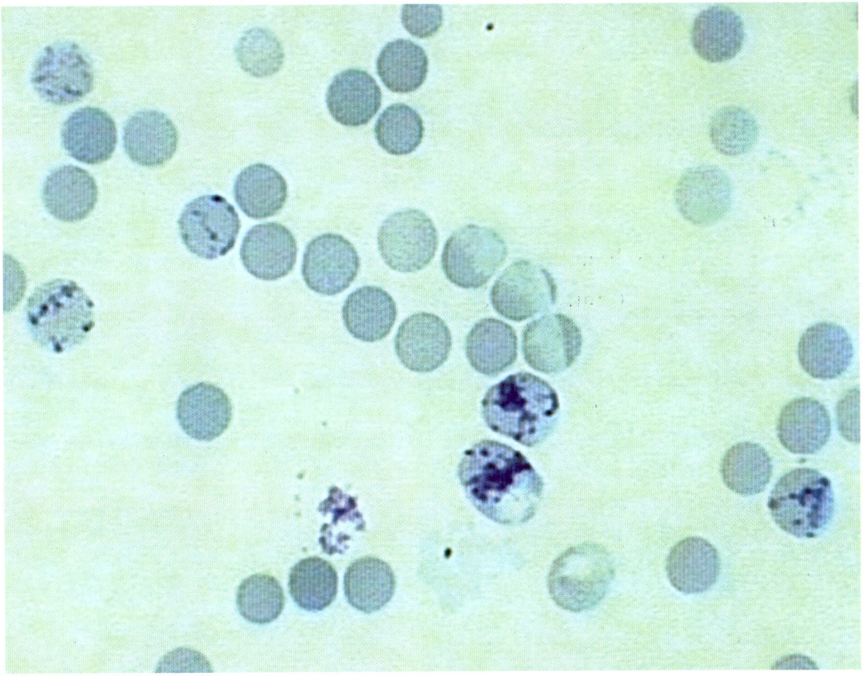

Fig. 3.1: Reticulocyte preparation of a patient with hemolytic anemia

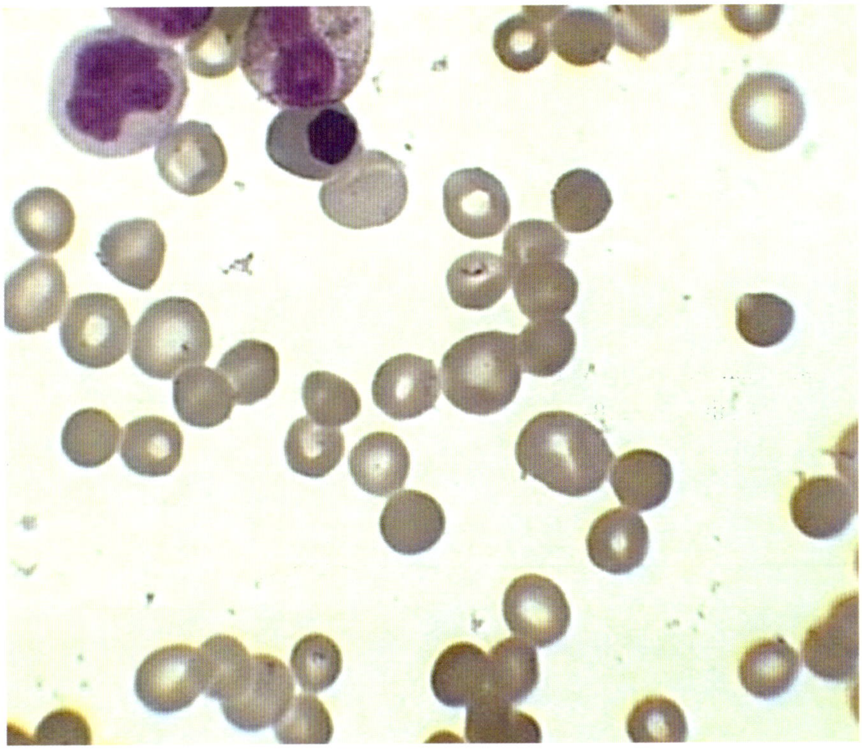

Fig. 3.2: Peripheral smear showing spherocytic red cells and nucleated RBC

- Cold agglutinin disease (Fig. 3.3)
- Acute alcoholism
- Hemoglobin C disease
- Hemolytic transfusion reactions
- Severe hypophosphatemia
- Acute oxidant injury: Hexose monophosphate shunt defect
- *Clostridium welchii* septicemia
- Following severe Burn injury. Of the above, autoimmune hemolytic anemia and hereditary spherocytosis are most common. The two can be further differentiated based on clinical history
- *Coombs test*: Sometimes spherocytes due to autoimmune hemolytic anemia may be associated with immune-mediated thrombocytopenia as in Evans syndrome.

b. *Hypochromic microcytes:* Peripheral smear with microcytic hypochromic cells along with general features of hemolysis are seen in the following:
   - Thalassemia (β-, α-thalassemias) including HbH disease (Fig. 3.4)
   - Hemoglobinopathy

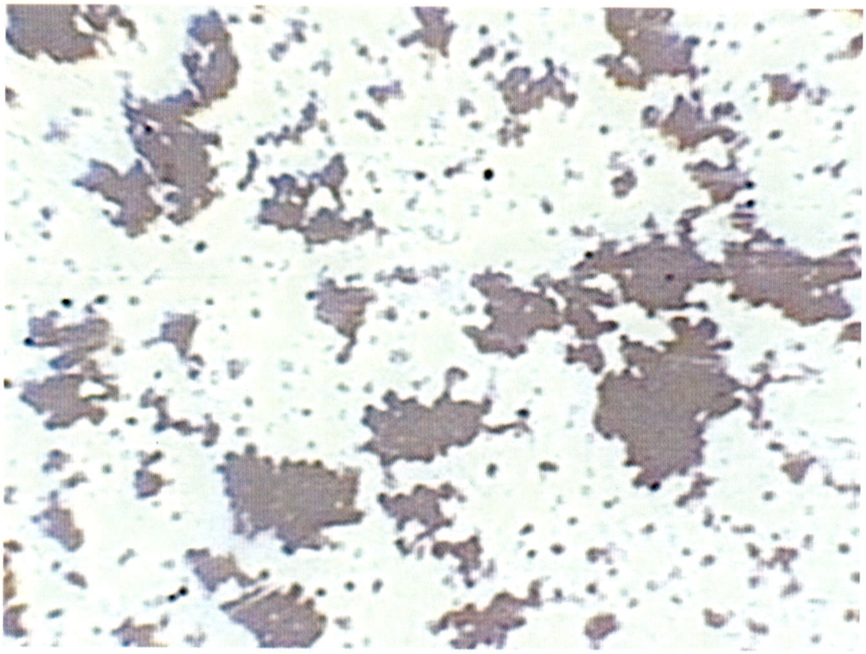

Fig. 3.3: Peripheral smear showing red cell agglutination seen in cold hemagglutinin disease

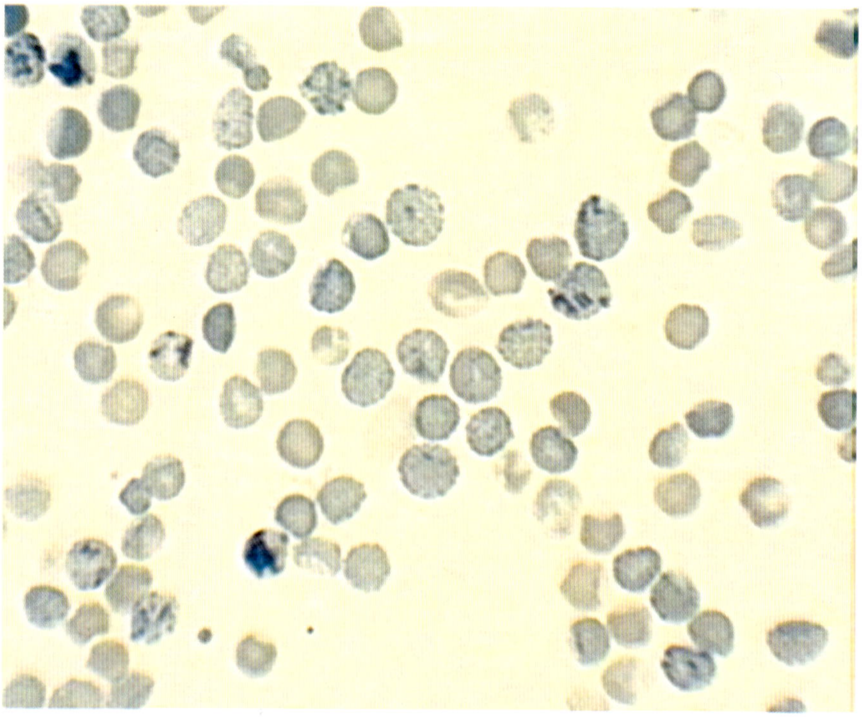

Fig. 3.4: HbH preparation showing golf-ball inclusions

- Sickle cell anemia
- β-thalassemia homozygous/hemoglobinopathies shows marked anisopoikilocytosis, basophilic stippling, target cells and nucleated RBC in addition to microcytic hypochromic cells (Fig. 3.5)
- *β-heterozygous thalassemia* shows microcytic hypochromic cells with basophilic stippling. Red cell indices show low MCV, high red cell count and normal red cell distribution unlike iron deficiency.
- *Sickle cell anemia:* This hemoglobinopathy is diagnosed by typical red cell sickles. It may or may not be associated with β-thalassemia trait which is suggested if surrounding cells are microcytic along with target cells (Fig. 3.6). Sometimes patients with sickle cells will show Howell-Jolly bodies due to autosplenectomy.
- The conclusive diagnosis of these is made on HPLC (Figs 3.16 to 3.29).

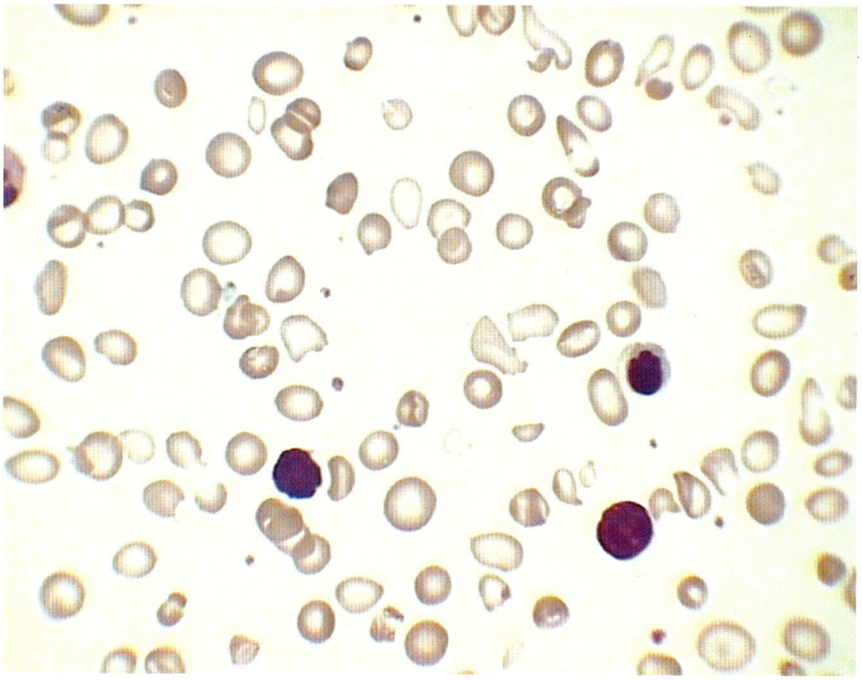

Fig. 3.5: Thalassemia major showing microcytic hypochromic cells, nucleated RBC and anisopoikilocytosis

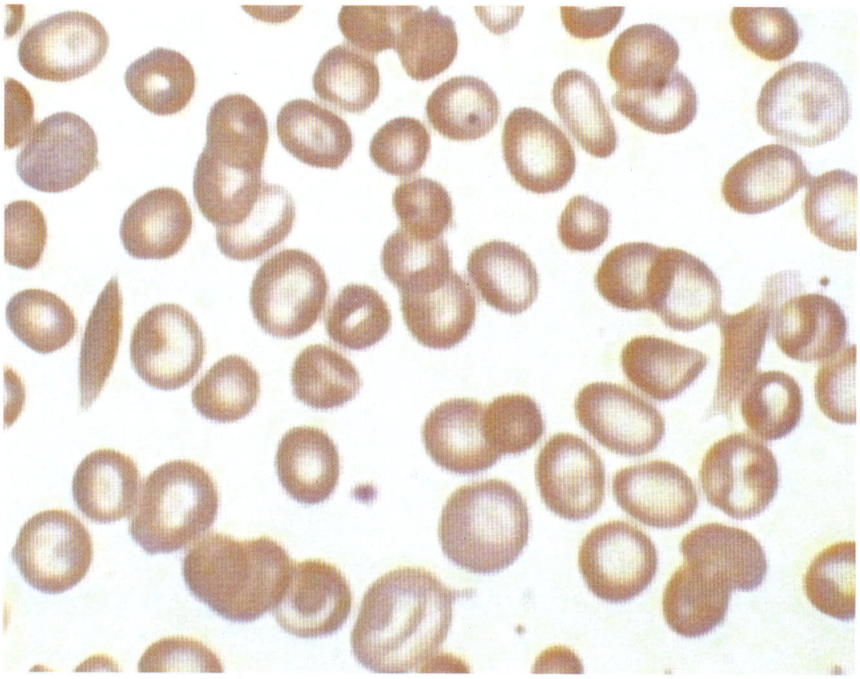

Fig. 3.6: HbS/β-thalassemia showing sickle cells, target cells and microcytic hypochromic cells

c. *Schistocytes (fragmented red blood cells) (Fig. 3.7):* These are typically seen in the following:
- Disseminated intravascular coagulation (DIC)
- Thrombotic thrombocytopenic purpura (TTP)
- Hemolytic uremic syndrome (HUS)
- Giant hemangioma
- Metastatic carcinoma
- Malignant hypertension
- Eclampsia (Toxemia of pregnancy)
- Vasculitis
- Prosthetic heart valve.

d. *Basophilic stippling (aggregated ribosomes) (Fig. 3.8):* This is typically seen in the following:
- Thalassemia
- Sideroblastic anemia
- In lead poisoning, peripheral smear shows coarse punctate basophilia.

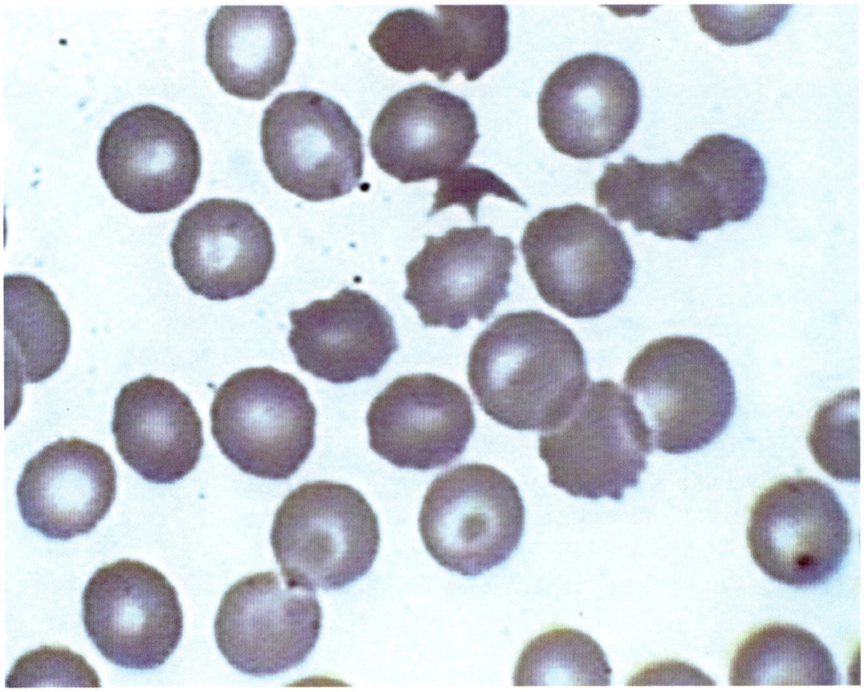

Fig. 3.7: Schistocyte

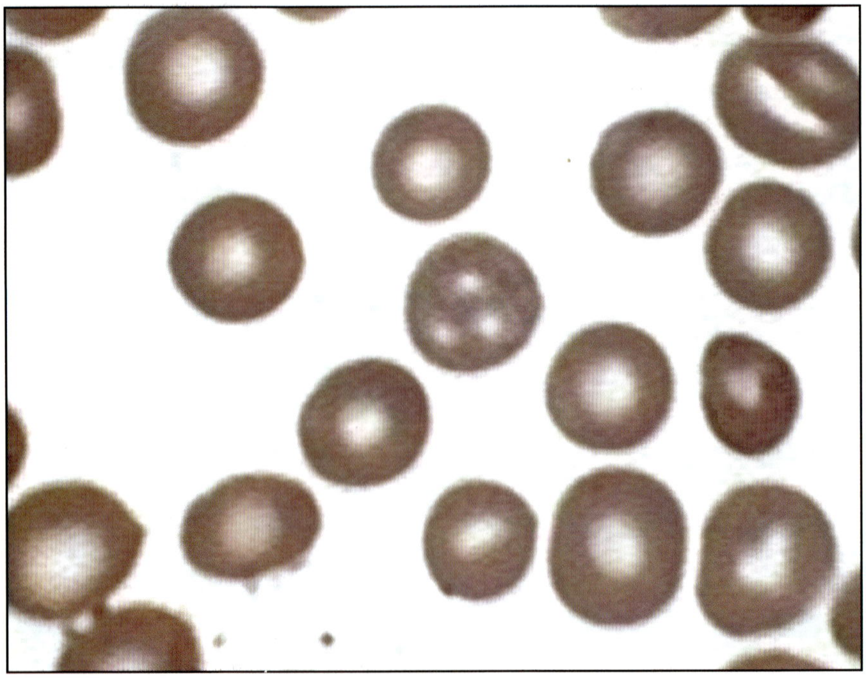

Fig. 3.8: Basophilic stippling

e. *Howell-Jolly bodies:* These are nuclear remnants which are seen as a nuclear remnants in the RBC (Fig. 3.9), typically seen in asplenic patient which may be due to:

- *Postsplenectomy:* In this case if Howell-Jolly bodies are not seen, it suggests the presence of accessory spleen.
- *Congenital asplenia:* In infants showing Howell-Jolly bodies in their RBC, congenital asplenia is suspected. This is associated with situs inversus.

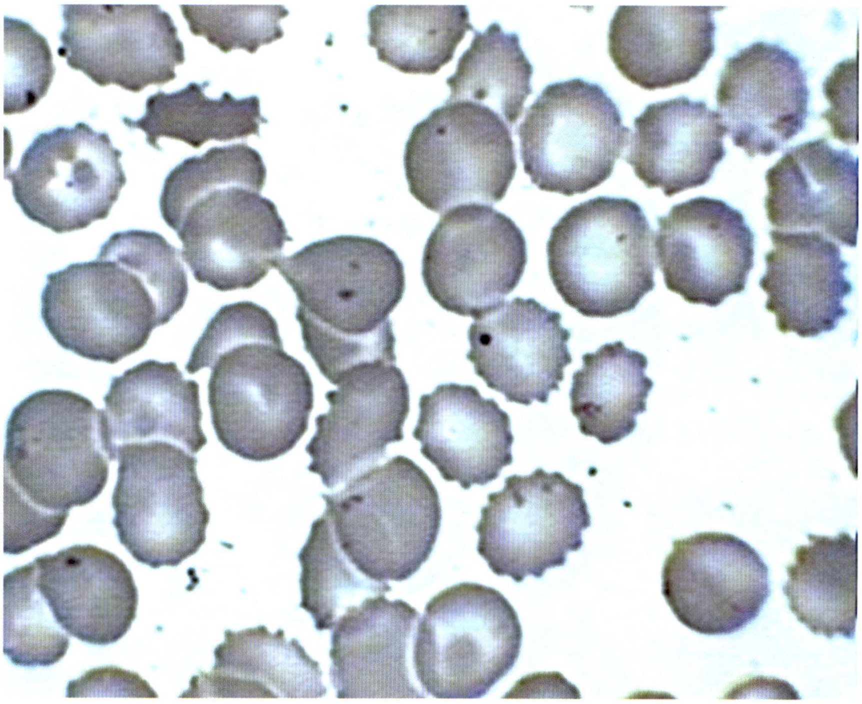

Fig. 3.9: Howell-Jolly body

DIAGNOSIS OF HEMOGLOBINOPATHIES

Hemoglobinopathies can be diagnosed with reasonable certainty with cation exchange. High performance liquid chromatography (HPLC) where different hemoglobins have different retention time. Given below are representative chromatographs of common hemoglobinopathies (Figs 3.10 to 3.23).

COMMON HIGH PERFORMANCE LIQUID CHROMATOGRAPHY (HPLC) PATTERNS (FIGS 3.10 TO 3.23)

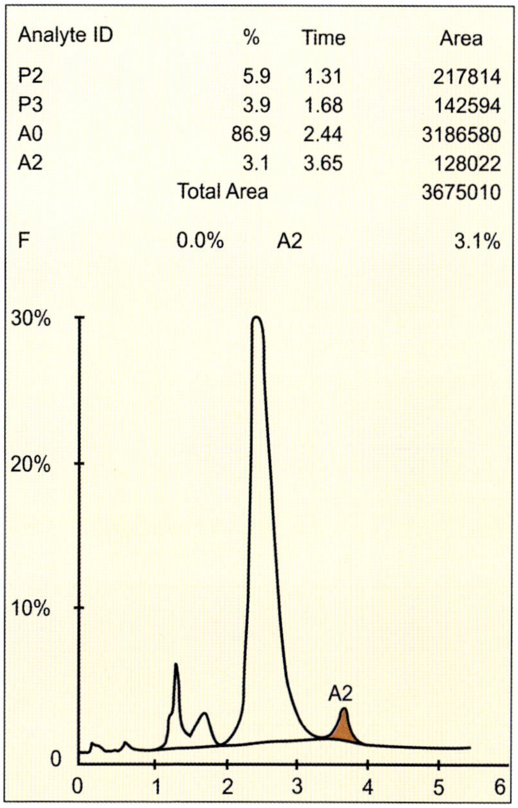

Fig. 3.10: Normal Hb HPLC

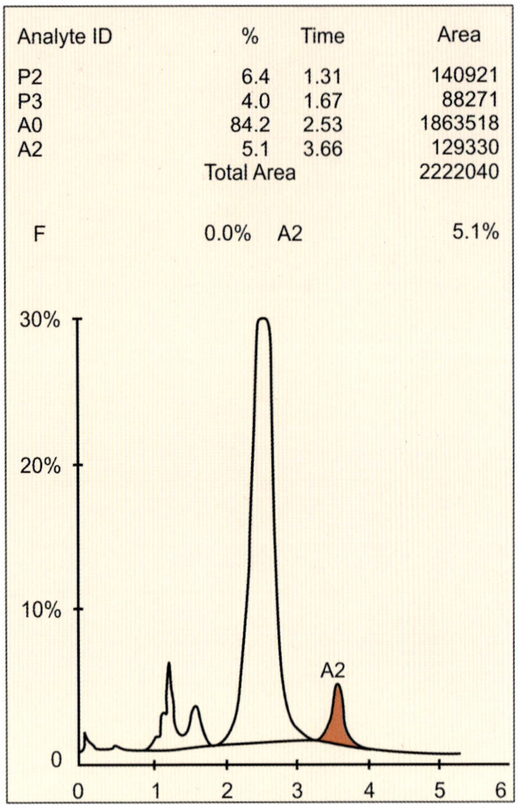

Fig. 3.11: Heterozygous β-thalassemia

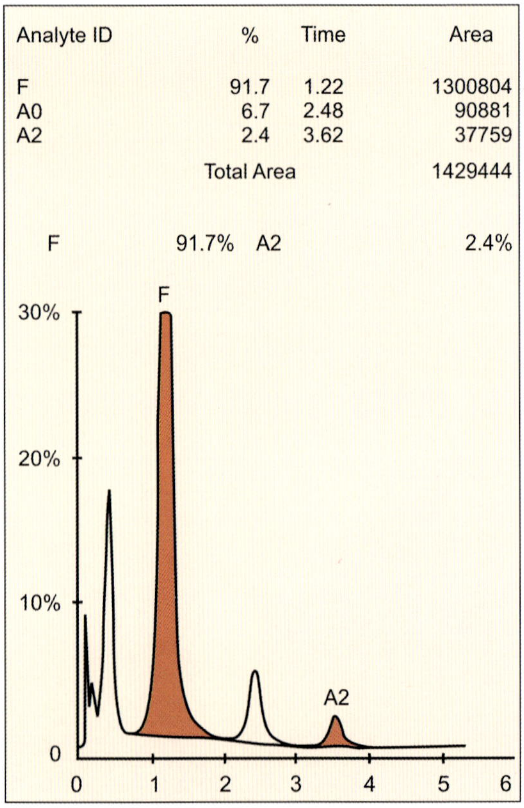

Fig. 3.12: Homozygous β-thalassemia (very high HbF)

Analyte ID	%	Time	Area
F	13.0	1.16	248374
P2	5.7	1.30	102888
P3	4.5	1.67	81451
A0	73.4	2.46	1319765
A2	3.3	3.61	63205
	Total Area		1815683

F 13.0% A2 3.3%

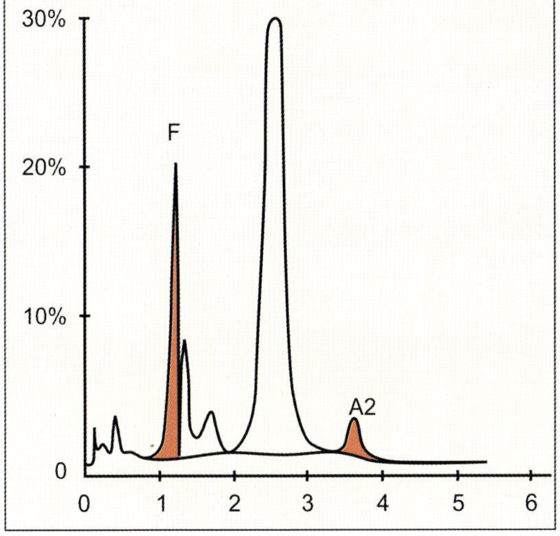

Fig. 3.13: Delta β-thalassemia (High HbF with normal HbA2)
Note: Red cell indices were suggestive of heterozygous β-thalassemia

Analyte ID	%	Time	Area
F	4.6	1.12	131136
P2	4.3	1.28	119084
P3	4.4	1.64	122414
A0	71.8	2.45	2011643
A2	9.3	3.45	292763
Unknown 1	5.4	3.59	150757
	Total Area		2827797

F 4.6% A2 9.3%

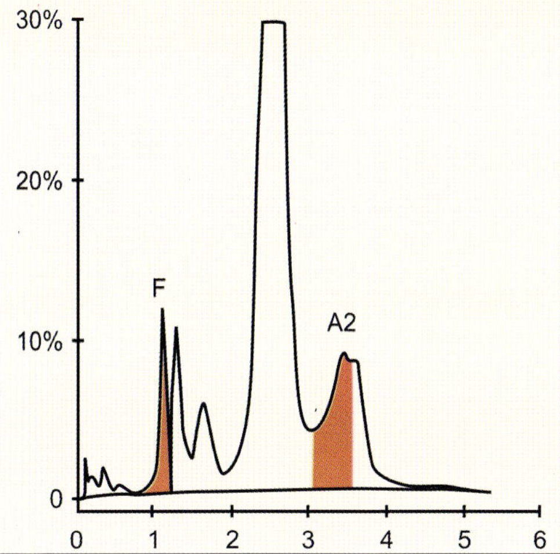

Fig. 3.14: Hb lepore (High HbA2 with hump in the A2 peak

Analyte ID	%	Time	Area
P2	6.0	1.29	184892
P3	5.1	1.70	157125
A0	62.1	2.46	1929732
A2	25.0	3.74	895972
	Total Area		3167721
F	0.0% A2		25.0%

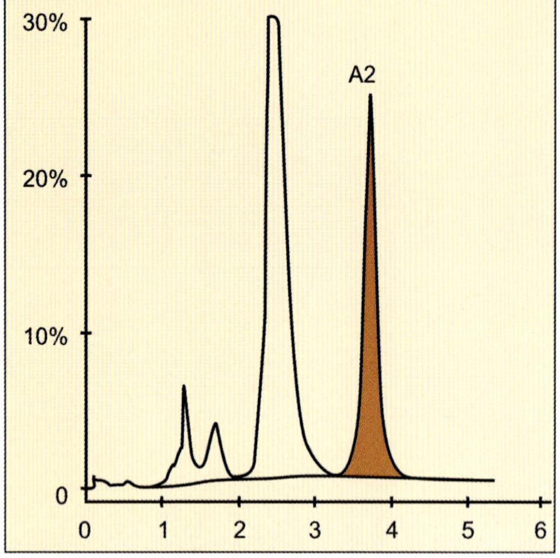

Fig. 3.15: Heterozygous HbE (two peaks HbA and HbA2)

Analyte ID	%	Time	Area
F	32.8	1.18	368996
Unknown 1	1.0	1.62	11110
P3	1.6	1.74	16899
Unknown 2	2.3	2.23	25064
A0	5.0	2.46	54296
A2	57.0	3.73	669394
	Total Area		1145759
F	32.8% A2		57.0%

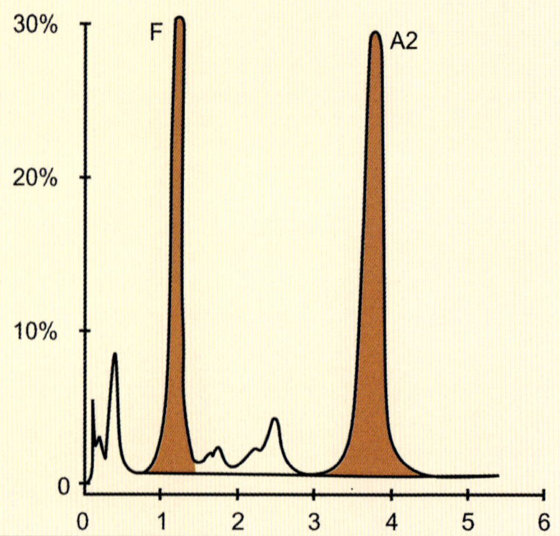

Fig. 3.16: HbE/β-thalassemia (high HbF and HbA2)

Analyte ID	%	Time	Area
P2	3.9	1.29	128107
P3	2.3	1.65	77577
A0	51.5	2.47	1712083
A2	3.6	3.66	132273
S-Window	38.6	4.42	1280829
	Total Area		3330889
F	0.0%	A2	3.6%

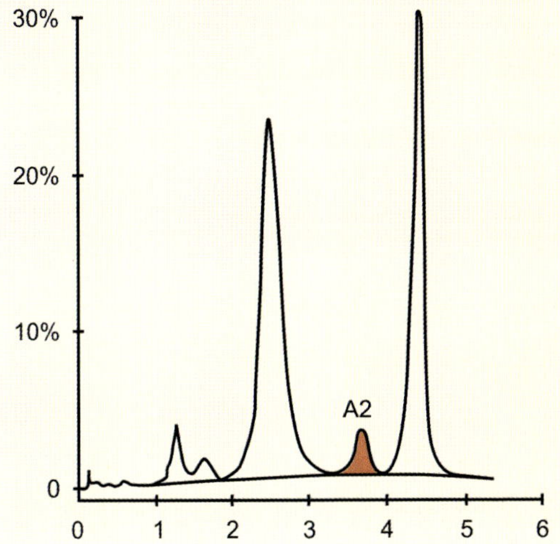

Fig. 3.17: Heterozygous HbS (two peaks HbA and HbS)

Analyte ID	%	Time	Area
F	20.0	1.19	459290
P3	0.5	1.61	10373
Unknown 1	2.3	2.28	49741
A0	4.3	2.46	94089
A2	4.6	3.66	110162
S-Window	68.6	4.40	1513803
	Total Area		2237458
F	20.0%	A2	4.6%

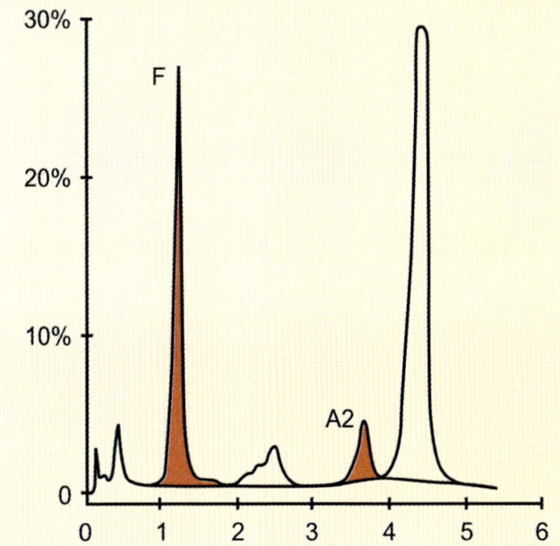

Fig. 3.18: Heterozygous HbS/β-thalassemia (high HbF)

Analyte ID	%	Time	Area
F	0.4	1.12	12020
P2	4.7	1.30	130452
P3	3.3	1.68	92456
A0	76.8	2.44	2143843
A2	1.9	3.64	61047
Unknown 1	0.6	4.55	17371
C-Window	11.5	4.88	321652
Unknown 2	0.7	5.02	18200
	Total Area		2797041
F	0.4% A2		1.9%

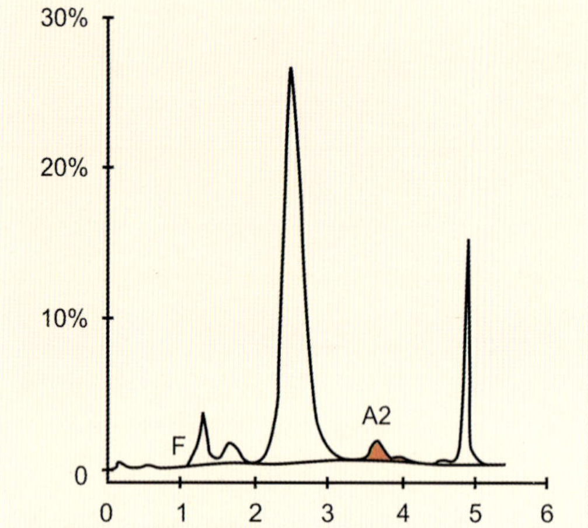

Fig. 3.19: Heterozygous HbC

Analyte ID	%	Time	Area
F	1.0	1.24	37698
P2	2.8	1.33	93049
P3	2.8	1.69	93522
Unknown 1	2.3	2.06	76189
A0	47.8	2.45	1614663
A2	3.3	4.40	121672
D-Window	40.0		1350829
	Total Area		3387622
F	1.0% A2		3.3%

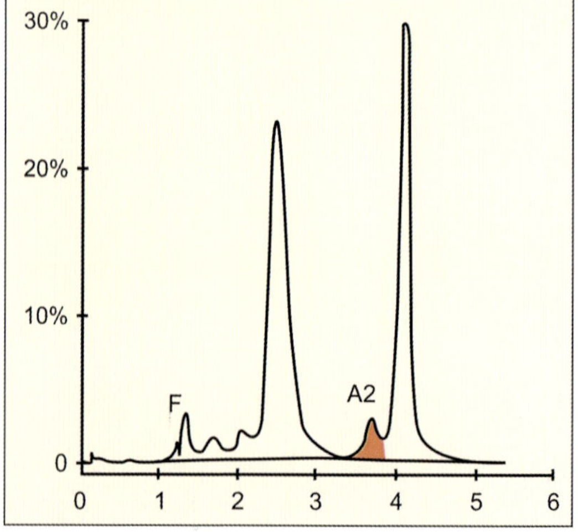

Fig. 3.20: Heterozygous HbD (two peaks HbA and HbD)

Analyte ID	%	Time	Area
F	2.6	1.16	76183
Unknown 1	0.3	1.91	8501
A0	1.4	2.08	38385
Unknown 2	0.9	2.30	25959
Unknown 3	0.7	2.93	19370
A2	3.6	3.68	107240
D-Window	44.2	4.06	1225317
B-Window	46.2	4.38	1279564
	Total Area		2780519
F	2.6%	A2	3.6%

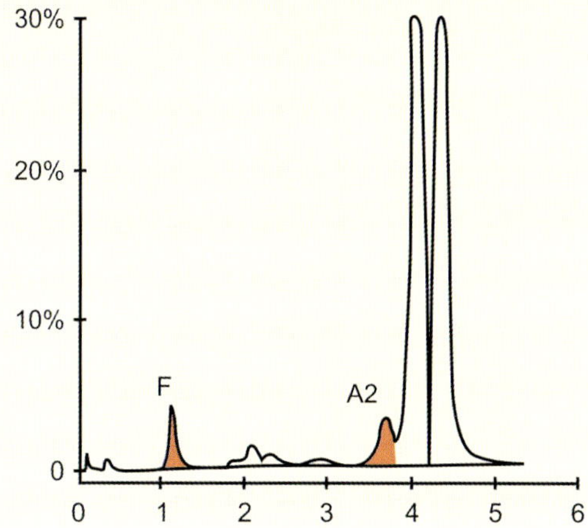

Fig. 3.21: Compound heterozygous HbD/HbS

Analyte ID	%	Time	Area
F	0.7	1.12	24225
P2	0.7	1.31	142359
P3	3.7	1.69	112130
A0	75.7	2.40	2309139
A2	5.6	3.67	179867
Unknown 1	8.4	4.70	257069
Unknown 2	1.3	4.83	39300
	Total Area		3063089
F	0.7%	A2	5.6%

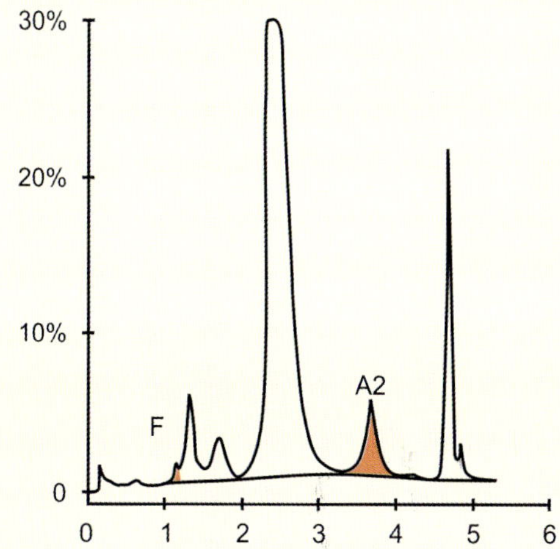

Fig. 3.22: HbQ India with heterozygous β-thalassemia [Unknown peak 1 (Q India) and High HbA2]

Analyte ID	%	Time	Area
F	0.5	1.24	5806
P2	2.2	1.36	22926
Unknown 1	0.3	1.54	2968
P3	2.4	1.72	24760
A0	92.6	2.40	956096
A2	2.0	3.64	21461
	Total Area		1034017
F	0.5%	A2	2.0%

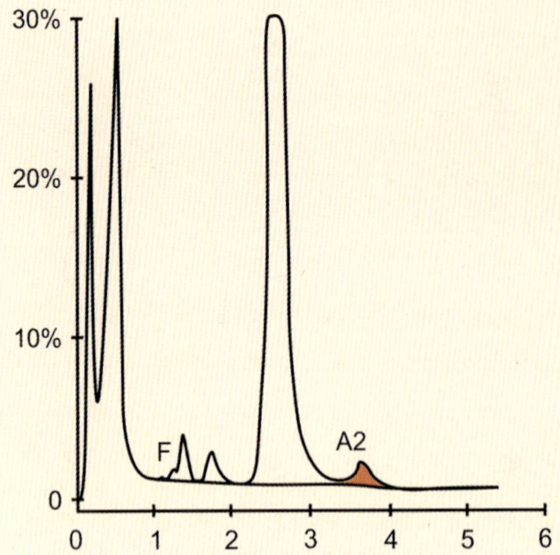

Fig. 3.23: HPLC tracing showing prerun peaks representing HbH and barts

CONGENITAL DYSERYTHROPOIETIC ANEMIA (CDA)

This is suspected when features of hemolysis are seen in a patient with anemia and hepatosplenomegaly and all tests for anemia are negative. Bone marrow shows marked dyserythropoiesis (Fig. 3.24). This is a rare form of chronic anemia with a varied clinical and hematological manifestations characterized by long standing anemia with ineffective erythropoiesis due to marked dyserythropoietic changes in the bone marrow (Fig. 3.25). The definitive diagnosis of this is made by characteristic morphological features of erythroblasts in electron microscopy.

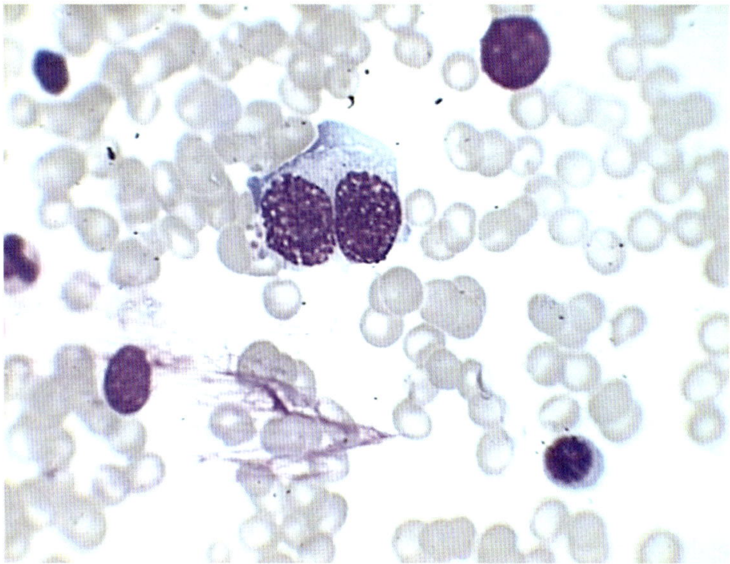

Fig. 3.24: Bone marrow of congenital dyserythropoietic anemia showing a binucleate erythroid cell

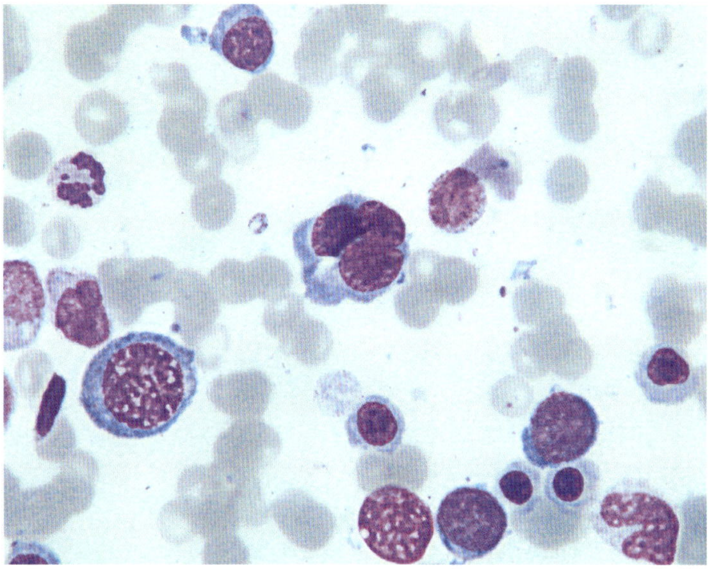

Fig. 3.25: Bone marrow of congenital dyserythropoietic anemia showing dyserythropoiesis

Clinical Features

See table 3.2.

Table 3.2: Clinical Features

Types	*Bone marrow*	*Blood picture*	*Inheritance*
I	Megaloblastic + intranuclear chromatin bridges	Macrocytic RBC	Recessive
II (HEMPAS)*	Bi/multinuclearity with, pluripolar mitosis	Normocytic RBCs, Lysis in acidified serum (not autologous serum)	Recessive
III	Giant erythroblasts with dominant multinuclearity	Macrocytic	Dominant, Sporadic

*Hereditary erythroblast multinuclearity with positive acidified serum (HEMPAS) test; commonest form, found in ~66% cases

Other Clinical Features

- Age of presentation variable; but usually in older children (>10 years). Can rarely present as neonatal jaundice and anemia
- Anemia—in type I, Hb 8.0–12.0 g/dL; type II anemia may be more severe, patient may be transfusion dependent. Type III (rare) anemia is mild/moderate
- Jaundice (2° to intramedullary RBC destruction)
- Gallstones
- Splenomegaly common.

Treatment

- Mostly unnecessary
- Blood transfusion and iron chelation as necessary
- Splenectomy not curative but may decrease transfusion requirements
- Type I may respond to high dose IFN-α; not recommended as routine therapy.

THALASSEMIA

β-Thalassemia Trait

- Carrier state
- Hb may be low but is not usually <10.0 g/dl
- Blood film: microcytic, hypochromic RBCs; target cells often present. Basophilic stippling especially in Mediterraneans
- HbA2 increased—provides useful diagnostic test for β-thalassemia trait.

β-Thalassemia Intermedia

- Denotes thalassemia major not requiring regular blood transfusion; more severe than β thalassemia trait but milder than β-thalassemia major
- Present with symptoms similar to β-thalassemia major but with only moderate degree of anemia
- Hepatosplenomegaly
- Iron overload is a feature
- Some patients are severely anemic (Hb ~6 g/dl) although not requiring regular blood transfusion, have impaired growth and development, skeletal deformities and chronic leg ulceration
- May require intermittent blood transfusion, iron chelation, folic acid supplementation and prompt treatment of infection, as for β-thalassemia major.

β-Thalassemia Major (Cooley's anemia)

- Presents in first year of life with transfusion dependent anemia and recurrent bacterial infection
- There is extramedullary hemopoiesis with hepatosplenomegaly and skeletal deformities
- Because of bone marrow expansion, there may be deformities of the skull with marked bossing and overgrowth of the zygomata, giving rise to the classical 'mongoloid facies' of β-thalassemia. These signs are associated with radiological changes, which include a lacy, trabecular pattern of the long bones and phalanges and a typical 'hair-on-end' appearance of the skull (Fig. 3.26)

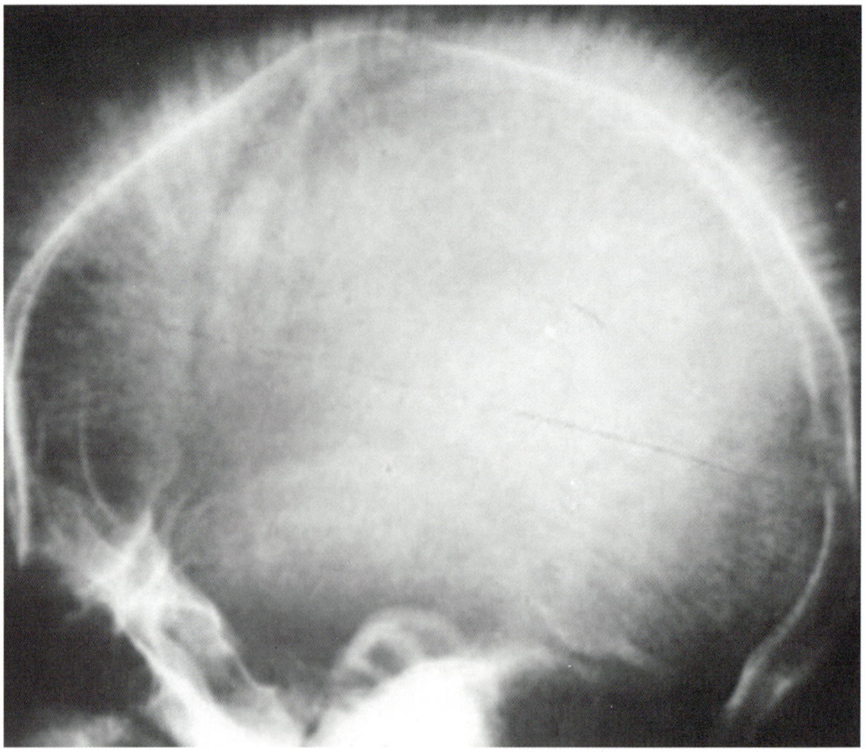

Fig. 3.26: X-ray skull lateral view showing expansion of marrow and hair-on-end appearance

- Marked anisopoikilocytosis, target cells and nucleated red cells
- Hb electrophoresis shows mainly HbF, HbA2 may be normal or mildly elevated.

Management

- Regular lifelong blood transfusion (every 2–4 weeks) to *suppress* ineffective erythropoiesis and allow normal growth and development in childhood
- Iron overload (*transfusion hemosiderosis*) is a major problem—damages heart, endocrine glands, pancreas and liver. Iron chelation therapy is routinely required starting after one year of regular transfusions (Fig. 3.27)
- Splenectomy may be of value (e.g. if massive splenomegaly or increasing transfusion requirements) but best avoided until after the age of five years due to increased risk of infection.
- Bone marrow transplantation has been carried out using sibling donor
- HLA-matched transplant is only curative.

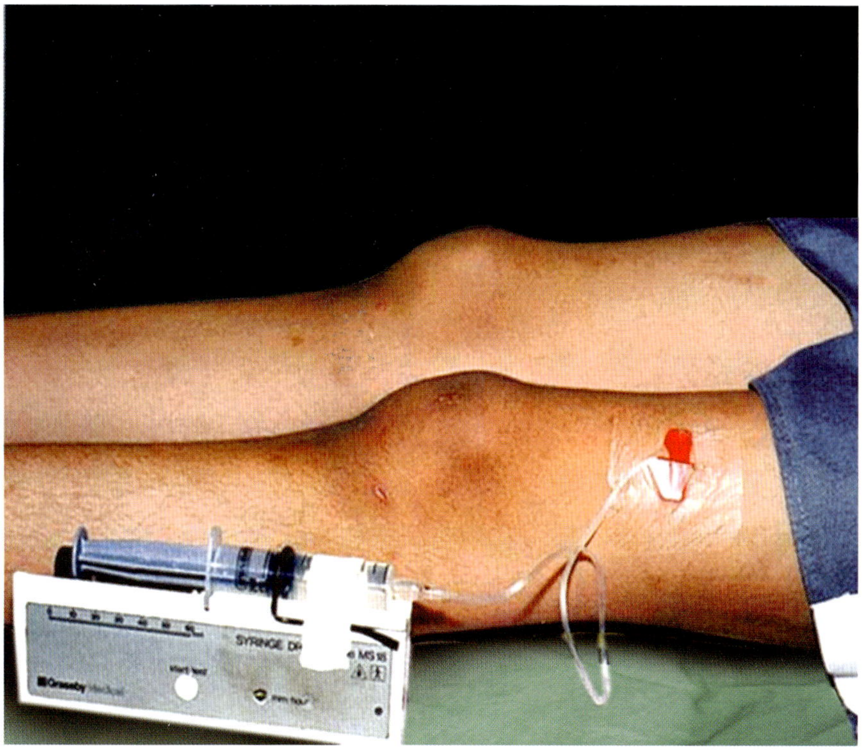

Fig. 3.27: Iron chelation therapy with desferroxamine being given by subcutaneous infusion pump to a patient of thalassemia major

HEREDITARY SPHEROCYTOSIS

Clinical Features

- Most common inherited RBC membrane defect characterized by variable degrees of hemolysis, spherocytic RBCs with increased osmotic fragility
- Usually autosomal dominant inheritance
- Abnormal RBC cytoskeleton: partial deficiency of spectrin, ankyrin, band 3 or protein 4.2
- Presents at any age
- Highly variable from asymptomatic to severely anemic, but usually there are few symptoms (Fig. 3.28). Well-compensated hemolysis
- Other features of hemolytic anemia may be present, e.g. splenomegaly, gallstones, mild jaundice (Fig. 3.29)
- Occasional aplastic crises occur, e.g. with parvovirus B19 infection
- Treatment is supportive folic acid and packed cell transfusion in severely affected
- Splenectomy is curative.

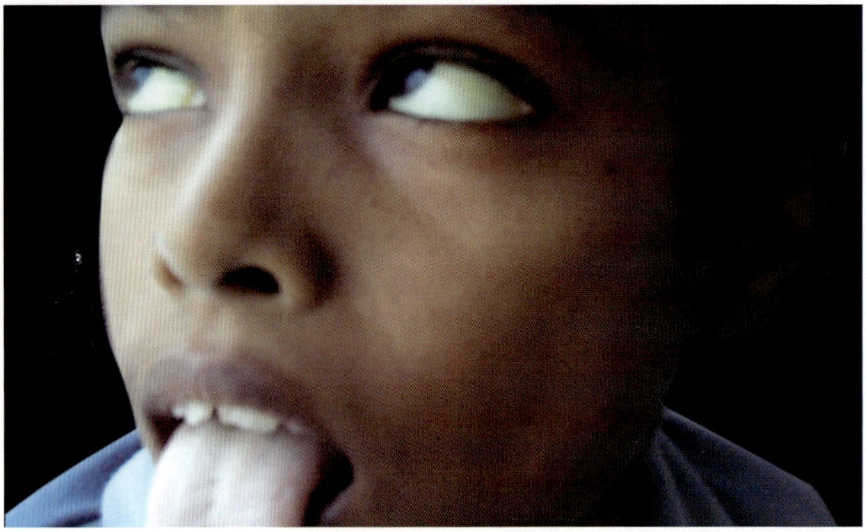

Fig. 3.28: Pallor and icterus in a patient of hereditary spherocytosis

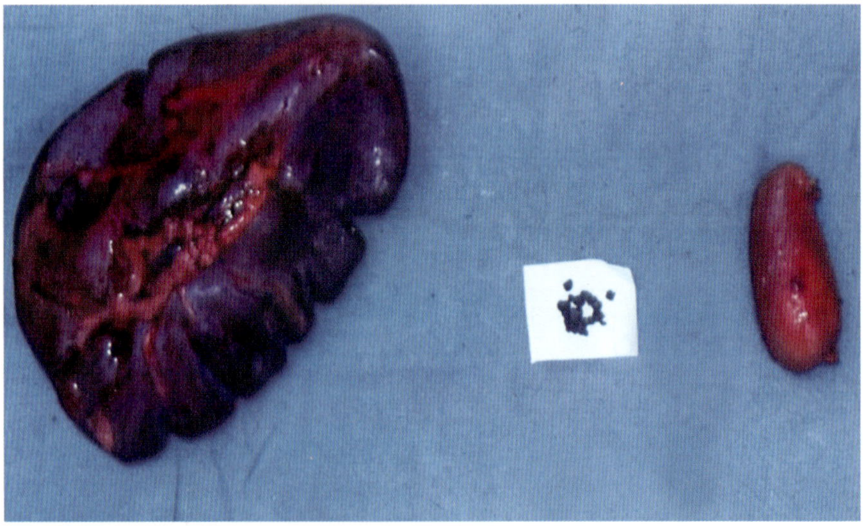

Fig. 3.29: Simultaneous splenectomy and cholecystectomy (with pigment gallstones) in a patient of hereditary spherocytosis

CHAPTER 4

Disorders of Platelets

CHAPTER OVERVIEW

- Thrombocytopenia
- Primary immune thrombocytopenia (ITP)
- Thrombotic thrombocytopenic purpura/HUS
- Platelet function defects
- Thrombocytosis

Disorders of platelets include thrombocytopenia, platelet function disorders and thrombocytosis.

THROMBOCYTOPENIA

Causes of Thrombocytopenia

Decreased Bone Marrow Production of Platelets

- *Marrow failure:* Aplastic anemia
- *Marrow infiltration:* Leukemias, myelodysplasia, myeloma, myelofibrosis, lymphoma, metastatic carcinoma
- *Marrow suppression:* Cytotoxic drugs and radiotherapy, other drugs (e.g. chloramphenicol)
- *Selective megakaryocytic:* Ethanol, drugs (phenylbutazone, co-trimoxazole; penicillamine), chemicals, viral infection (e.g. HIV, parvovirus)
- *Nutritional deficiency:* Megaloblastic anemia
- *Hereditary causes (rare):* Fanconi's syndrome, congenital megakaryocytic hypoplasia, absent radii (TAR) syndrome.

Increased Destruction of Platelets

Immune

- Primary immune thrombocytopenia
- Associated with other autoimmune states SLE, CLL, lymphoma
- *Drug-induced:* Heparin, gold, quinidine, quinine, penicillins, cimetidine, digoxin
- *Infection:* HIV, other viruses, malaria
- Post-transfusion purpura
- Neonatal alloimmune thrombocytopenia.

Nonimmune

- DIC
- TTP/HUS
- Kasabach-Merritt syndrome
- Congenital/acquired heart disease
- Cardiopulmonary bypass.

Platelet Sequestration

Hypersplenism

Dilutional Loss of Platelets

- Massive transfusion
- Exchange transfusion

Hereditary Thrombocytopenia

Wiskott-Aldrich syndrome, May-Hegglin anomaly, Bernard-Soulier syndrome.

PRIMARY IMMUNE THROMBOCYTOPENIA (ITP)

Thrombocytopenia may be due to a number of causes which include reduced production, as in aplastic anemia, increased destruction as in ITP, hypersplenism or leukemia etc. Bone marrow can help differentiate between aplastic anemia from other causes of thrombocytopenia.

Based on bone marrow examination, two types of pictures can be seen (Figs 4.1A and B):

1. *Megakaryocytic thrombocytopenia:* This shows a cellular bone marrow with normal erythroid and myeloid components and prominence of megakaryocytes. This is seen typically in immune-mediated thrombocytopenia where a large number of young megakaryocytes

are seen (Fig. 4.1A). Young magakaryocytes differ from mature megakaryocytes by being smaller and having rounded contours, deep blue cytoplasm and single lobed nucleus (Fig. 4.1B). Mature megakaryocytes are large and have lilac-colored cytoplasm with multilobed nucleus. Sometimes cultures of young megakaryocytes are also seen. This prominence of megakaryocytes occurs as a response of megakaryocytes to thrombopoietin which increases in thrombocytopenia.

Megakaryocytic thrombocytopenia (Presence of thrombocytopenia and megakaryocytes in BM) can be seen in megaloblastic anemia, hypersplenism, ITP, SLE, DIC, HUS, TTP and myelodysplastic syndrome. Sometimes, in ITP, there may be associated normoblastic erythroid hyperplasia due to associated iron deficiency.

2. *Amegakaryocytic thrombocytopenia:* This is best diagnosed on a bone marrow biopsy and is characterized by marked paucity of megakaryocyte in a cellular marrow with normal erythroid and myeloid precursors. It is important to know that sometimes in children the megakaryocytes are tightly adherent to the underlying periostium thereby being falsely absent on bone marrow aspirate. However, in such cases, bone marrow biopsy shows presence of megakaryocytes. Typically amegakaryocytic thrombocytopenia occurs due to thiazide diuretics, and estrogen, etc.

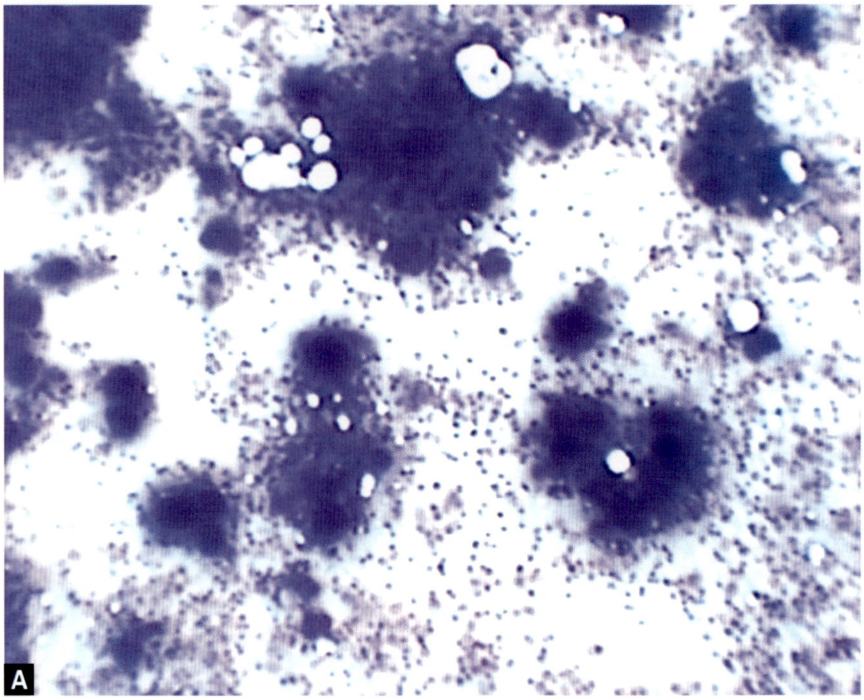

A

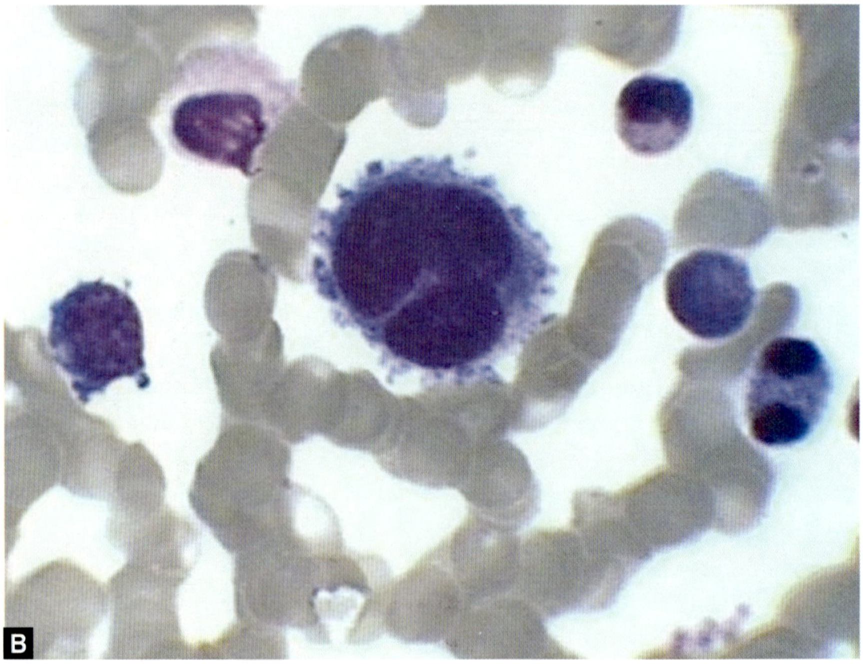

B

Figs 4.1A and B: (A) Bone marrow from a case of ITP (10X) showing marked prominence of megakaryocytes; (B) Bone marrow from a case of ITP (oil) showing young megakaryocytes with round contours and deep blue cytoplasm

Post-splenectomy changes in ITP:
ITP patients are often subjected to splenectomy. A complete splenectomy shows the following typical features in a peripheral smear. There is presence of large number of Howell-Jolly bodies (remnants of RNA in cytoplasm), target cells and thrombocytosis (Fig. 4.2). In case, these features are not present, in post-splenectomy smear, possibility of accessory spleen must be considered. Due to this, the patient may not respond to splenectomy till the accessory spleen is also removed.

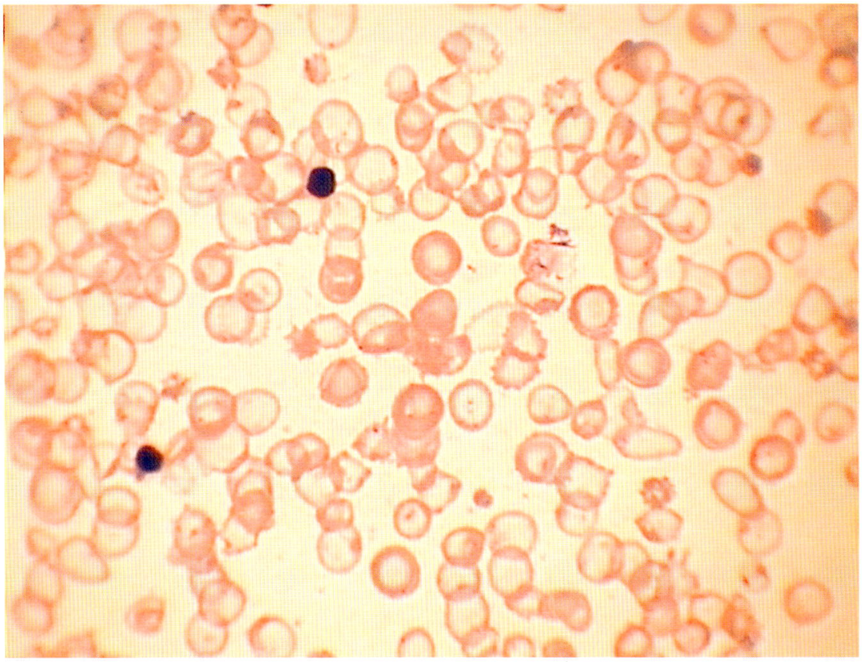

Fig. 4.2: ITP with splenectomy (Howell-Jolly bodies)

Clinical Features

- Usually presents with hemorrhagic manifestations like petechie, purpura, epistaxis, menorrhagia or bleeding gums but may occasionally be detected in an asymptomatic adult patient on a routine blood test (Fig. 4.3)

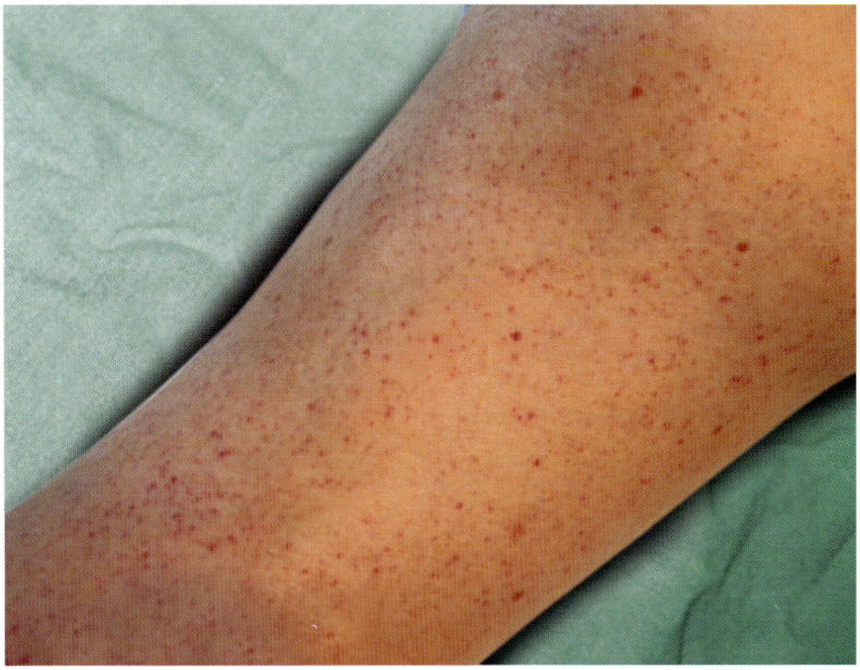

Fig. 4.3: Widespread petechiae and purpura in a classical case of primary immune thrombocytopenia

- Intracranial bleeds occur in <1 percent (associated with platelet count <10 x 10^9/L) (Fig. 4.4)
- Commonest in young adults
- Patient may have microcytic hypochromic anemia secondary to iron deficiency due to blood loss (Fig. 4.2)
- The natural history of childhood cases is acute in 90 percent and usually follows a self-limiting course without treatment. They are often associated with a history of previous viral illness and complete resolution may be expected within three months.
- In adults, a chronic course is usual and spontaneous resolution is rare (<5%).

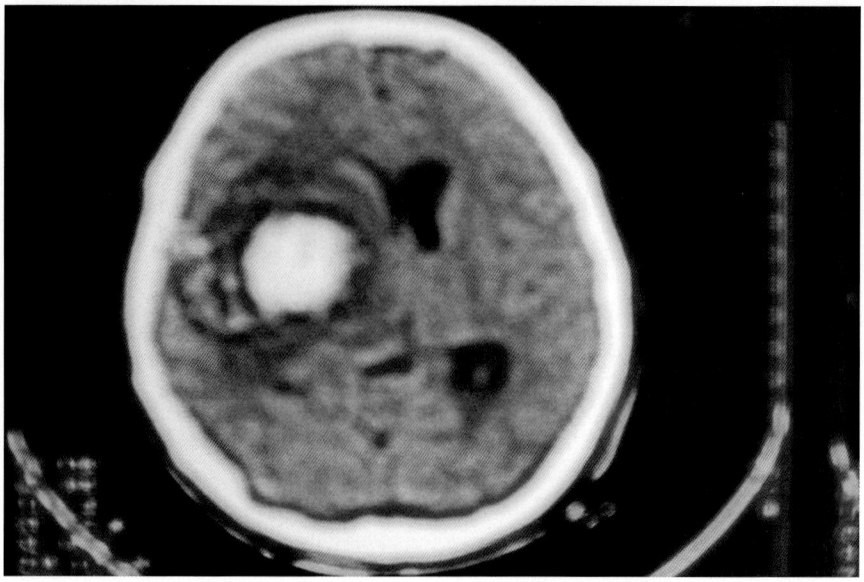

Fig. 4.4: CT scan—head showing intracranial bleeding in a patient with ITP

Treatment of ITP

- No need to treat mild compensated ITP (>30 × 10^9/L) unless hemorrhagic manifestations
- The initial treatment options include IVIG, anti-D and prednisolone
  - *Prednisolone:* First-line therapy for most patients, slow tapering to minimal doses. Initial dose should be at least 1 mg/kg/day. If no response by two to three weeks, it should be tapered off.
  - *IVIG:* Effect often rapid (within 4 days) but usually transient and lasts ~3 weeks. The cost of this therapy limited its use.
  - *Anti-D:* It can be used with a dose of 75 μg/kg. It should be used in nonsplenectomized and Rh+ ve patients.
- The best second-line treatment is splenectomy. Splenectomy should be done in patients who fail to respond to prednisolone or require prednisolone >10 mg/d to maintain acceptable platelet count
- 60 to 80 percent of patients achieve at least a partial response to splenectomy
- Immunosuppressive agents (azathioprine, vincristine, cyclophosphamide) and Rituximab may be used in patients who have failed to achieve an adequate response to splenectomy or in whom splenectomy is contraindicated.

THROMBOTIC THROMBOCYTOPENIC PURPURA/HUS

The classic pentad of symptoms that comprise the syndrome of TTP include:

- Microangiopathic hemolytic anemia (MAHA)
- Thrombocytopenia
- Neurologic symptoms
- Fever
- Renal dysfunction

MAHA resulting from fragmentation of red cells in the microvasculature is a sine qua non of this disorder. The presence of schistocytes on peripheral smear (Fig. 4.5) is the most characteristic laboratory finding.

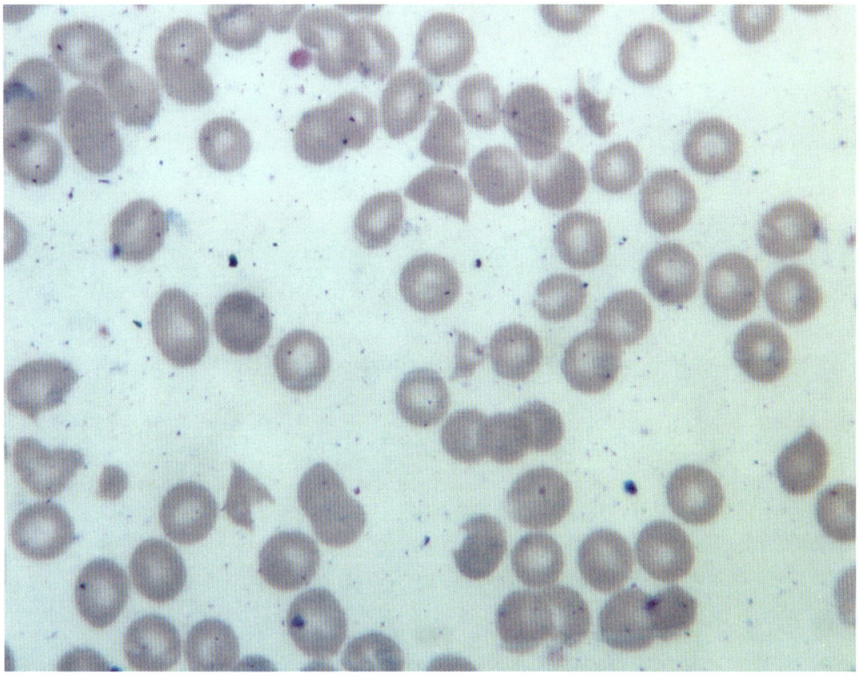

Fig. 4.5: Peripheral smear showing schistocytes in patient with TTP

PLATELET FUNCTION DEFECTS

Sometimes patients present with peticheal hemorrhages with normal platelet counts. These may be due to platelet function defects or capillary defects like Henoch-Schönlein purpura (this generally has a hand and glove distribution). The inherited platelet function defects include the following:

- *Bernard-Soulier syndrome:* Thrombocytopenia may be observed in platelet function defects like Bernard-Soulier syndrome. This can be best picked up on a peripheral smear examination where large platelets, nearly the size of small lymphocytes are seen (Figs 4.6 and 4.7).

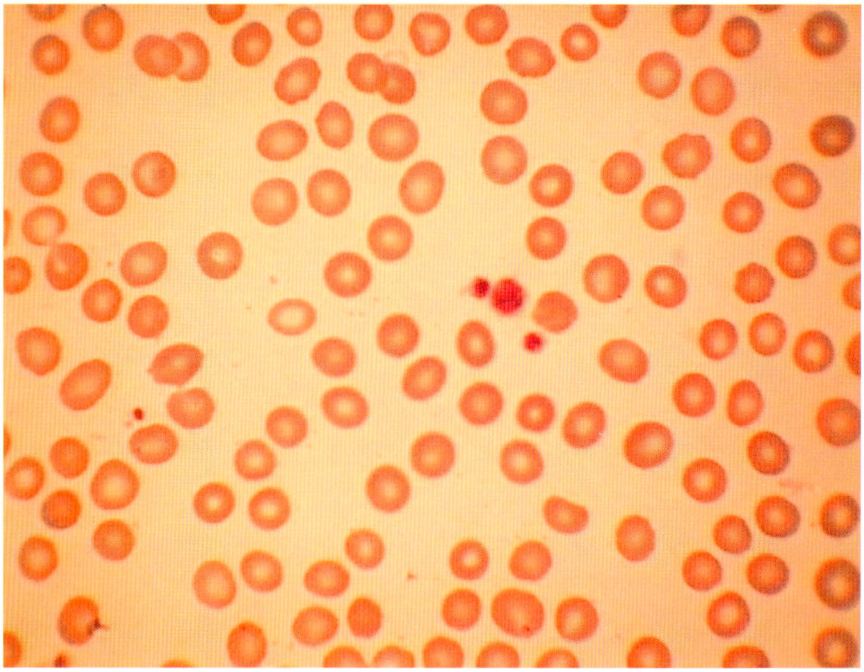

Fig. 4.6: Peripheral smear from a case with Bernard-Soulier syndrome showing a large platelet

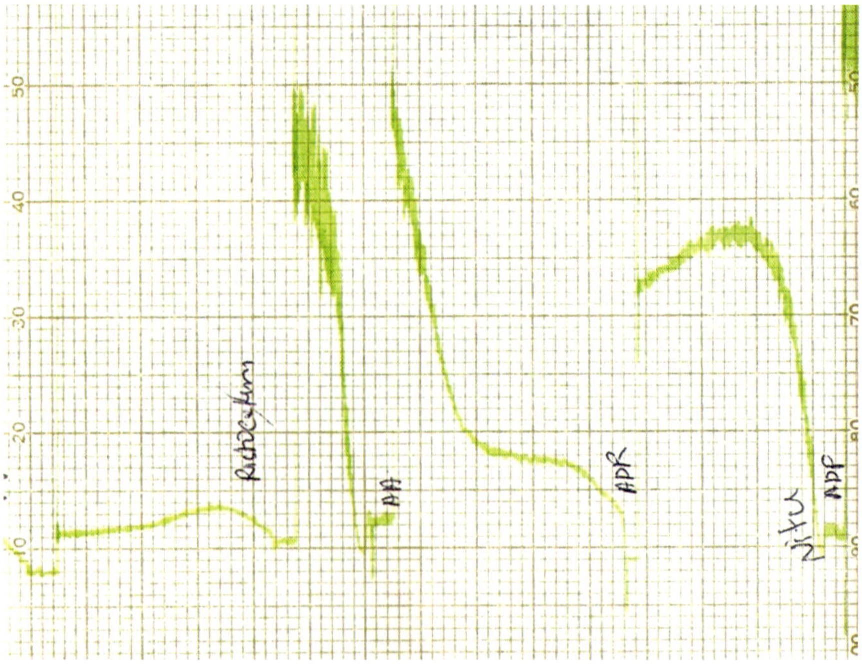

Fig. 4.7: Bernard-Soulier syndrome: Absent aggregation with ristocetin and normal with other agonists

- *Glanzmann's thrombasthenia (GT):* A fresh fingerprick smear can be used to diagnose GT. Presence of single platelets with absence of any platelet aggregate suggests GT. It is important to remember here that single platelets are often seen in an EDTA peripheral smear but never in a fresh fingerprick smear unless patient has Glanzmann's thrombasthenia (Fig. 4.8).

Clinical Features

- Mucocutaneous bleeding (skin, nose, gums, gut) with a positive family history (though not always found)
- All autosomal recessive. Carriers asymptomatic
- Clinically the bleeding symptoms are similar but may be other clinical features to distinguish the syndromes
- Menorrhagia may be troublesome. Bleeding in Glanzmann's may be severe and life-threatening.

THROMBOCYTOSIS

Persistent elevation of platelet count more than 4.5 lakh/cumm, is thrombocytosis (Fig. 4.9). It may be secondary to reactive changes to infections, iron deficiency, postoperative, postsplenectomy or as part of myeloproliferative disorders. Elevation of platelet counts in the absence of above disorders makes one suspect essential thrombocythenia (Fig. 4.9).

Treatment

No treatment is necessary for reactive thrombocytosis. In primary thrombocytosis, prophylactic use of antithrombotic agents has not been well delineated. In general, platelet-lowering agents have been recommended for high-risk patients (all adults) with an increased cardiovascular risk, have a previous history of thrombosis, or who are older than 60 years. Cytoreductive therapy like hydroxyurea can be used to reduce the platelet count.

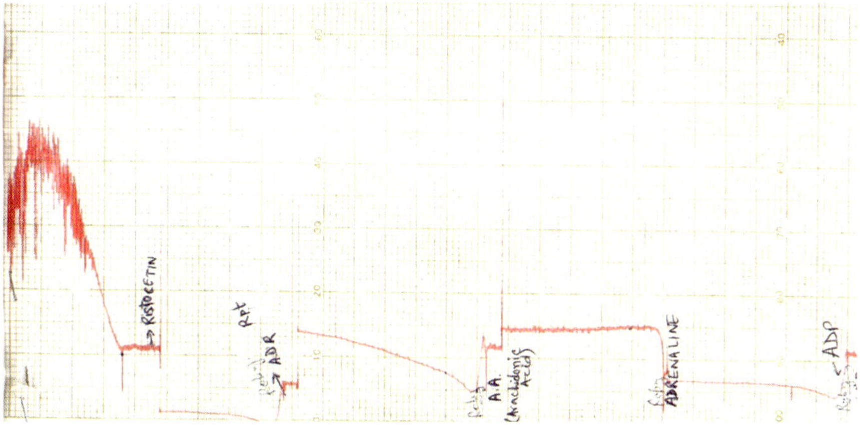

Fig. 4.8: Glanzmann's thrombasthenia: Normal aggregation with ristocetin and absent with ADP, adrenaline and arachidonic acid

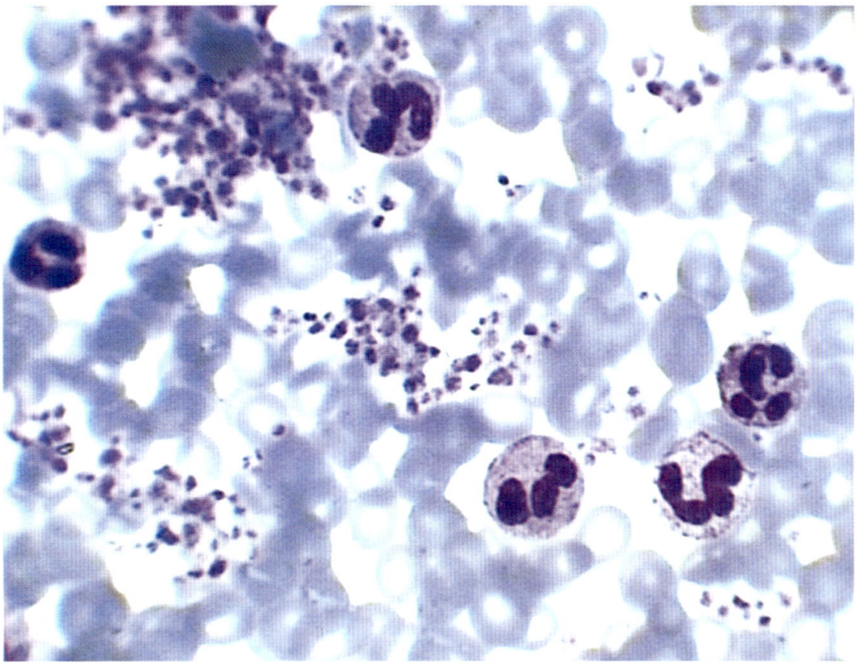

Fig. 4.9: Peripheral smear showing marked thrombocytosis

CHAPTER 5

Acute Leukemia

CHAPTER OVERVIEW

- Acute leukemia
- Acute lymphoblastic leukemia (ALL)
- Blast morphology
- Acute myeloid leukemia (AML)
- Biphenotypic leukemia
- Acute myeloblastic leukemia (AML) with multilineage dysplasia
- AML/MDS: Occupation related or therapy related

Leukemia is a disease resulting from the clonal neoplastic (tumor like) proliferation of the hematopoietic cells. As major site of hematopoiesis is the bone marrow, most leukemias begin in the bone marrow, spill over into the blood and finally involve organs like liver, spleen and lymph nodes. Depending on the stage of development of the cells mainly affected and the course of the disease, they may be classified into acute or chronic. Depending on the main cell type involved, they may be divided into lymphoid or non-lymphoid (i.e. myeloid) (Flow chart 5.1) and thus, leukemias may be broadly into:

- *Acute/chronic:* Depending on duration and progression of disease
- *Lymphoid/myeloid:* Depending on cell of origin

Flow chart 5.1: Classification of leukemia

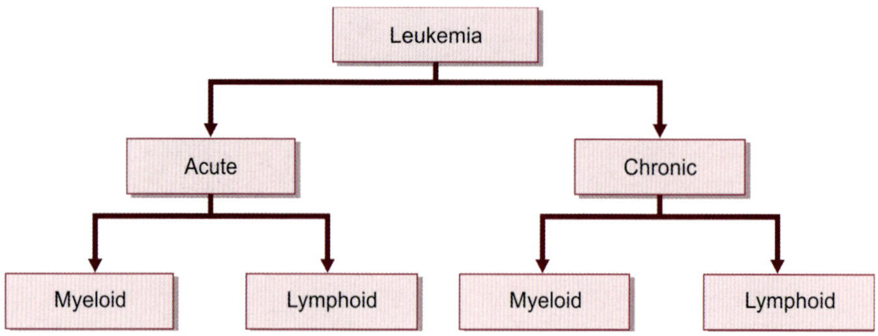

Rarely, the disease process may involve really primitive totipotent stem cells giving rise to mixed biphenotypic leukemias (both lymphoid and myeloid). More commonly, it is the white blood cells and their precursors which are involved. However, there are types of leukemias where precursors of red cells (erythroblasts) or of platelets (megakaryocytes) are involved.

ACUTE LEUKEMIA

Acute leukemia can be of two types:

- Acute lymphoblastic leukemia (ALL)
- Acute myeloblastic leukemia (AML)

ALL vs AML

Though all blasts (whether myeloid or lymphoid) are similar in appearance being large cells with high N : C ratio and opened up chromatin pattern, there are subtle morphological changes between the two. In general, lymphoblasts tend to be smaller, have coarser chromatin pattern and a very high N:C ratio. Nucleoli if present, number from one to two. Myeloblasts on the other hand are larger, have slightly more abundant cytoplasm along with a fine chromatin pattern. Nucleoli may number from two to five. The cytoplasm may show granules, Phi bodies or Auer rods which are pink-rod shaped structures (Figs 5.1A and B).

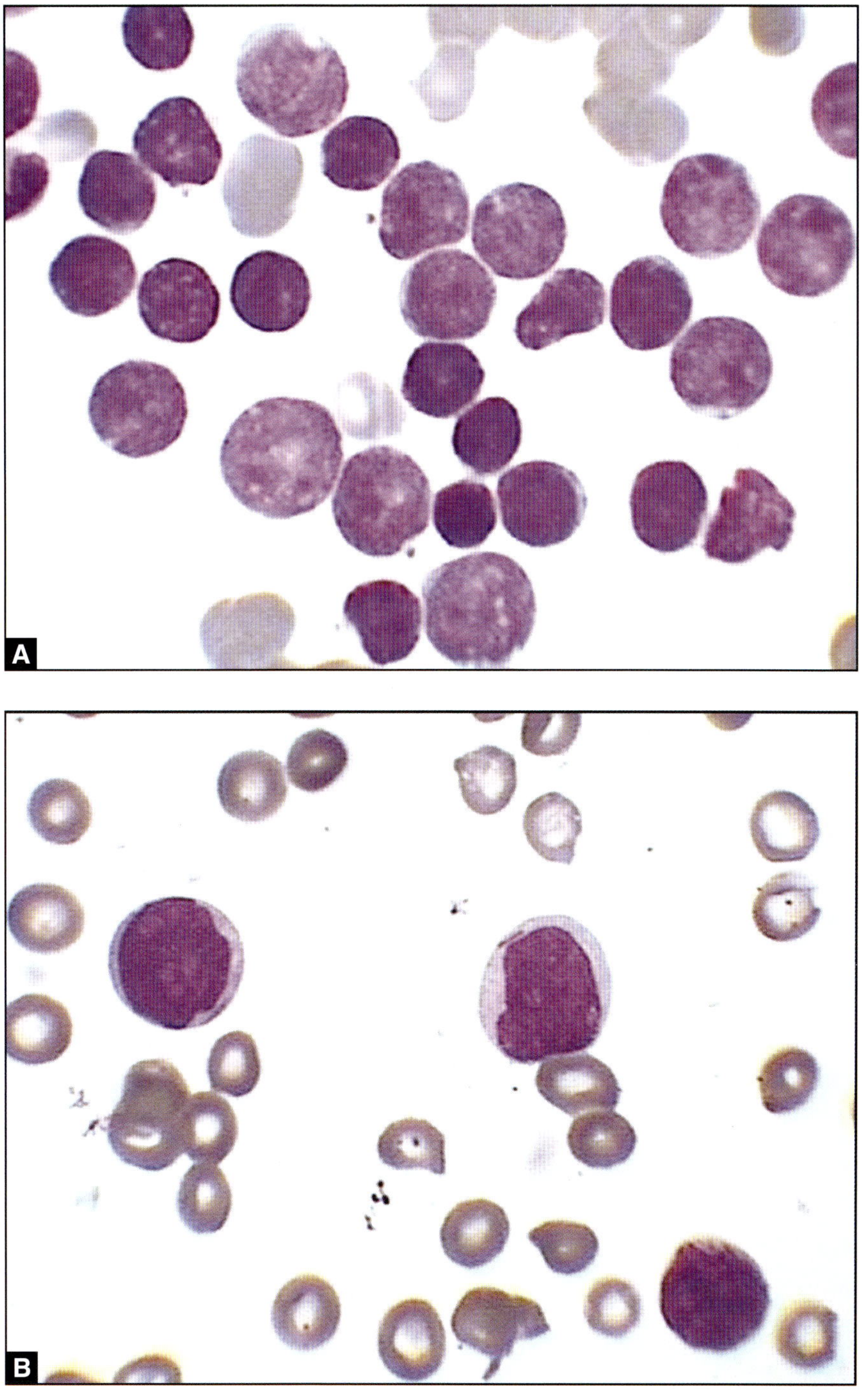

Figs 5.1A and B: (A) Acute lymphoblastic leukemia: Scant cytoplasm; (B) Acute myeloblastic leukemia (AML): Auer rod seen

ACUTE LYMPHOBLASTIC LEUKEMIA (ALL)

Acute lymphoblastic leukemia (ALL) comprises 80 percent of the acute leukemias of childhood. The peak incidence is between three and seven years of age. It comprises approximately 20 percent of adult acute leukemias.

Clinical Features

- *Acute presentation usual:* Often critically ill due to effects of bone marrow failure
- Symptoms of anemia: Weakness, lethargy, breathlessness, lightheadedness and palpitations
- *Infection:* Particularly chest, mouth, perianal, skin (*Staphylococcus, Pseudomonas*, HSV, *Candida*)
- *Hemorrhage:* Purpura, menorrhagia and epistaxis, bleeding gums, rectal, retina
- Signs of leukostasis, e.g. hypoxia, retinal hemorrhage, confusion or diffuse pulmonary shadowing
- Mediastinal involvement occurs in 15 percent specially in T-lineage ALL and may cause SVC obstruction (Fig. 5.7)
- CNS involvement occurs in six percent at presentation and may cause cranial nerve palsies especially of facial VII nerve, sensory disturbances and meningism
- Signs include widespread lymphadenopathy in 55 percent, mild-to-moderate splenomegaly (49%), hepatomegaly (45%) and orchidomegaly.

BLAST MORPHOLOGY

The French, American and British (FAB) classification of subtyping of acute leukemia was designed in 1982 and is commonly used. It is based on the type of blast cells predominating in the marrow and blood. These are of three types: L1, L2, L3. The characteristics of blasts in each subtype are given below:

L1 Blasts (Fig. 5.2)

These have the following characteristics:

- Small (twice the diameter of a red cell)
- High nuclear cytoplasmic ratio
- Nucleus regular in shape
- Nucleoli if seen, are small and inconspicuous.

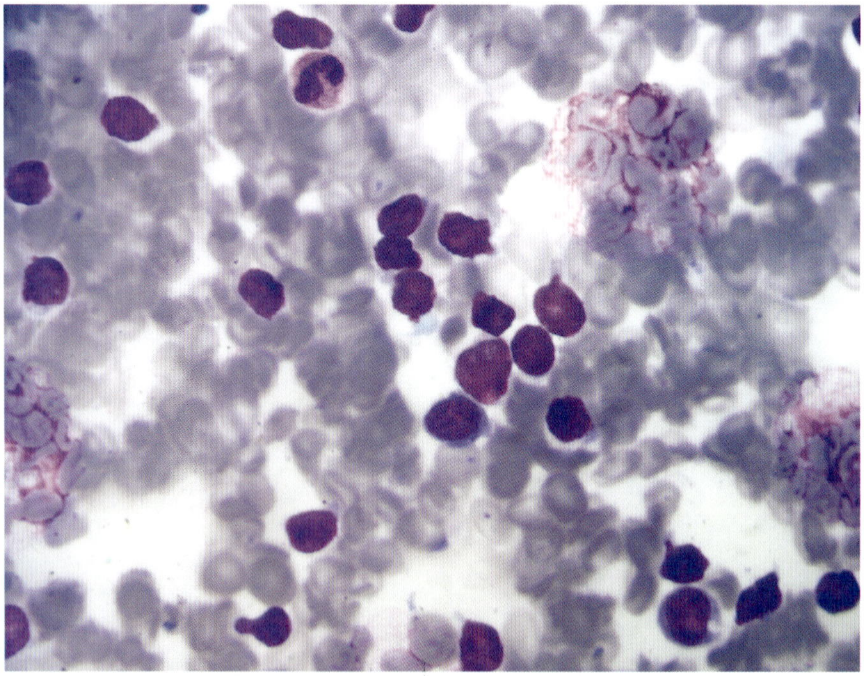

Fig. 5.2: Acute lymphoblastic leukemia:L1 blast

L2 Blasts (Fig. 5.3)

These have the following characteristics:

- Blasts are larger and heterogeneous
- Nuclei are irregular in shape with clefting in folding and indentation
- Nucleoli usually present and are large.

L3 Blasts (Fig. 5.4)

These have the following characteristics:

- Blasts are large and homogeneous
- N:C ratio is lower than in L1-ALL
- Nucleus is regular
- Prominent nucleoli
- Strongly basophilic cytoplasm
- Prominent cytoplasmic vacuolation.

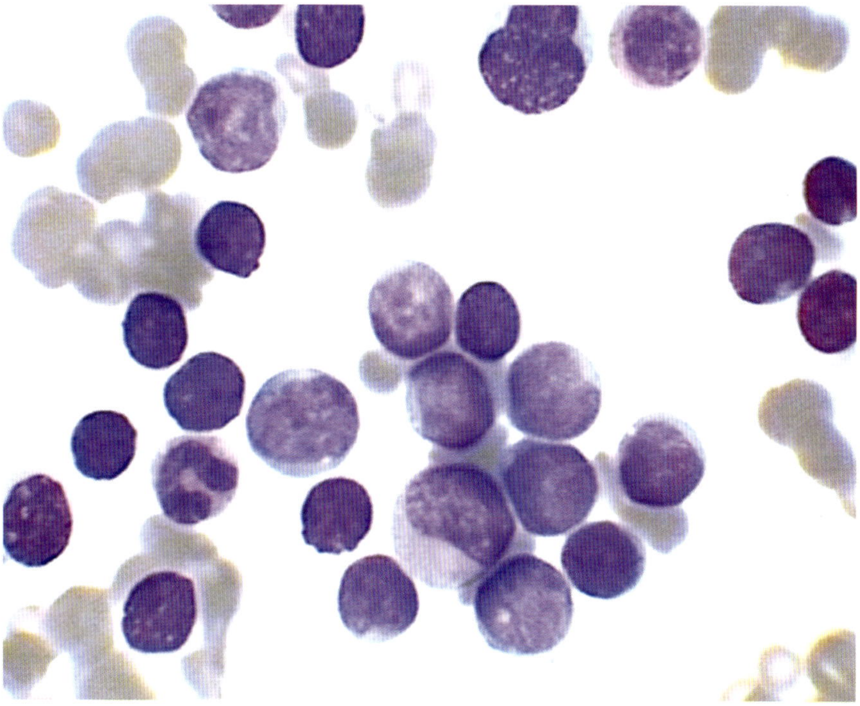

Fig. 5.3: Acute lymphoblastic leukemia (ALL): L2 blast (Giemsa)

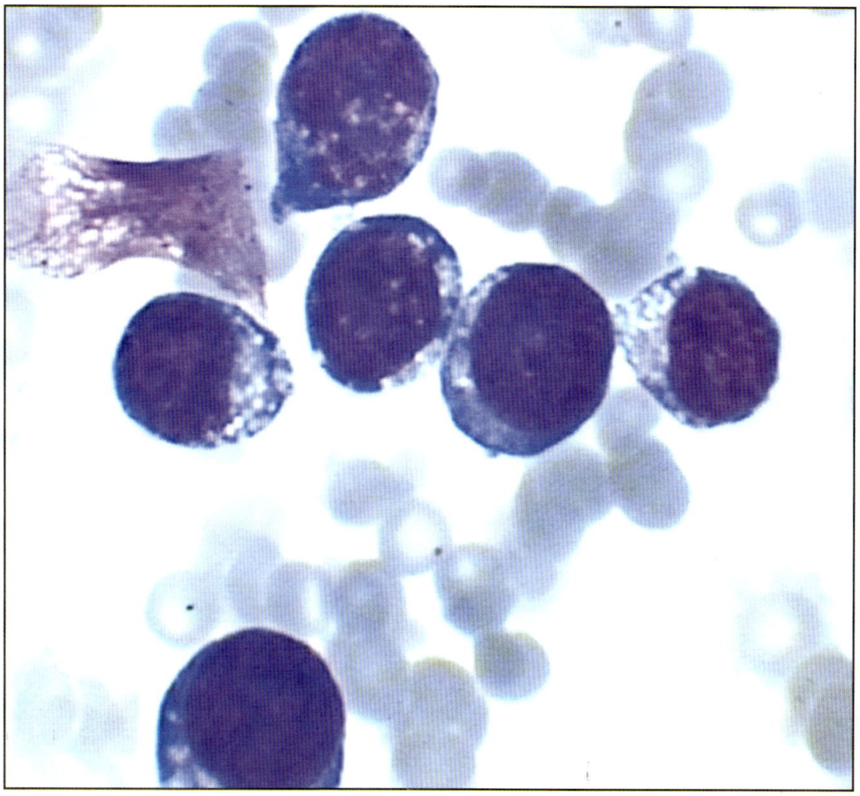

Fig. 5.4: Acute lymphoblastic leukemia (ALL): L3 blast showing vacuoles in cytoplasm (Giemsa)

Diagnosis

This is based on peripheral smear examination and blood counts, bone marrow findings, cytochemistry, immunophenotyping and molecular studies.

Blood and Peripheral Smear

- The total WBC count is often raised but may be normal or low
- Anemia, thrombocytopenia and neutropenia are common due to bone marrow failure
- The peripheral smear shows presence of immature cells, i.e. the blasts which may be of L1, L2, or L3 morphology.

Note: Sometimes it becomes difficult to differentiate ALL from NHL with spill. In such cases, it is important to look at hemoglobin and platelet counts. In acute leukemia, they are generally low whereas in most cases of NHL they may be normal. Clinically, duration of illness in acute leukemias is generally <6 months whereas in NHL it is >6 months. However in some cases of NHL, Hb and platelet count may be low. In such cases, immunophenotyping/immunohistochemistry may be helpful in differentiating between the two.

Bone Marrow

The bone marrow shows presence of blasts (<25% of bone marrow cells) the morphology of which may be suggestive of lymphoid origin. However, for more definitive diagnosis one needs to resort to cytochemisty.

Cytochemistry: The following special stains help in diagnosis:

- PAS—Lymphoblasts (of B-lineage) show block positivity for PAS (Fig. 5.5)
- Acid phosphatase—Strong polar positivity may be seen T-lymphoblasts
- Myeloperoxidase
- Sudan black lymphoblasts do not show any positivity
- Nonspecific esterase: It may show polar positivity in T lymphoblast.

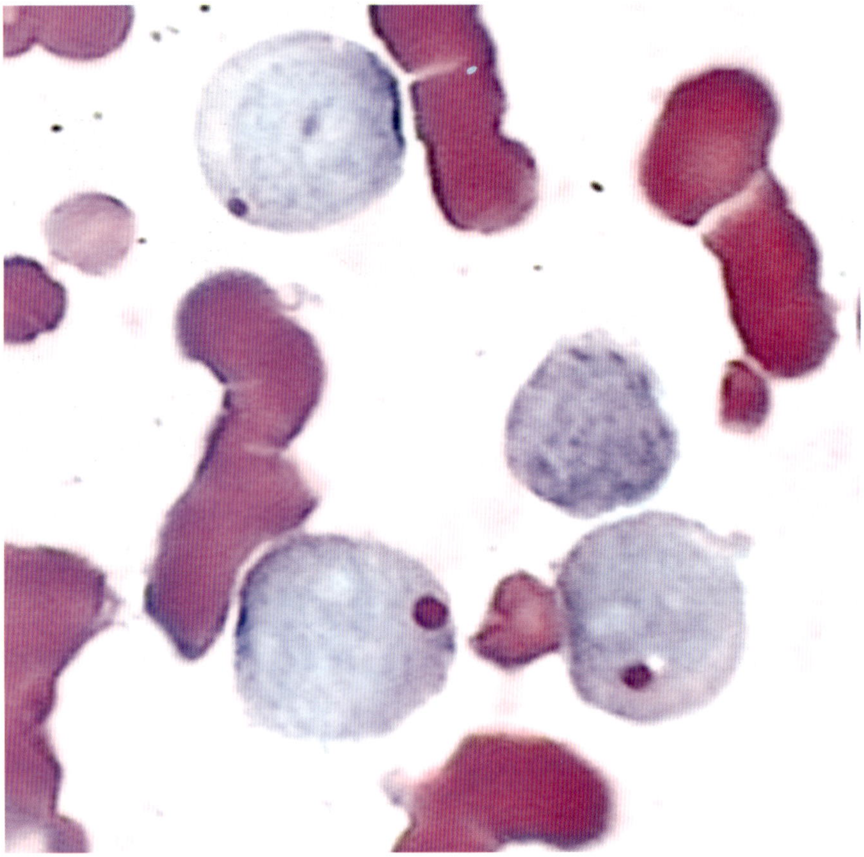

Fig. 5.5: PAS: Block positivity in ALL

Large Granular Lymphocytic Leukemia

This is a type of acute leukemia which arises from large granular lymphocytes (LGL)/Natural Killer cells (NK cells). The latter are derived from common lymphoid progenitor cells and have lifespan of a few days to a few weeks. Mature NK cells in peripheral blood constitute 15 percent of all lymphocytes and are not seen in marrow (<1% of lymphocytes). They are responsible for non MHC dependant cytotoxicity.

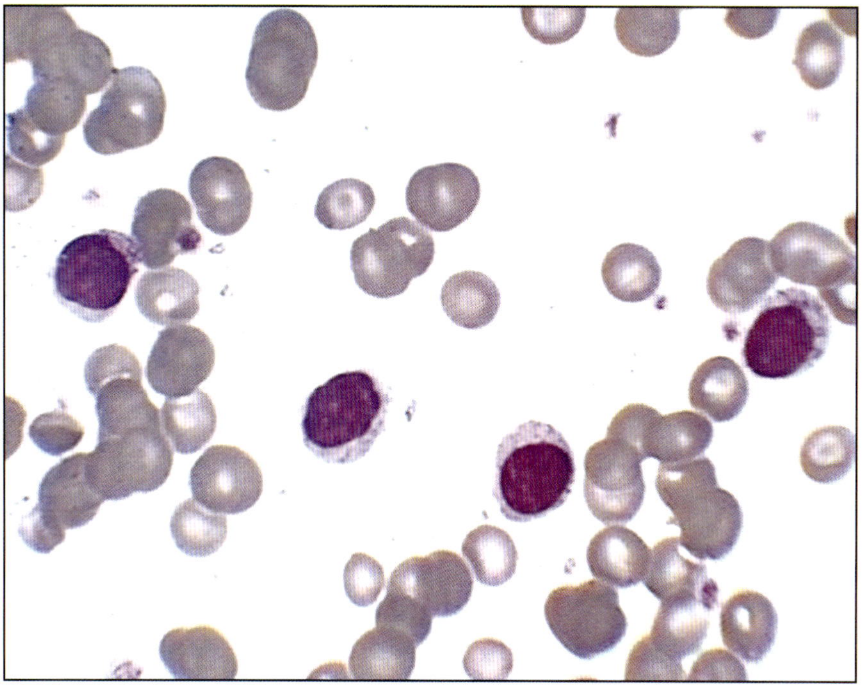

Fig. 5.6: Large granular cell leukemia cell

Morphology of Large Granular Lymphocytes (Fig. 5.6)

- Large sized lymphocytes
- Round or indented nuclei
- Condensed chromatin
- Prominent nucleoli
- Cytoplasmic granules (Primary lysosomes).

Treatment for ALL

It consists of five contiguous phases:

1. *Remission induction* using vincristine, prednisolone, daunorubicin and asparaginase to achieve complete remission; more intensive induction using more anthracycline improves leukemia-free survival.
2. *CNS prophylaxis* generally combines cranial irradiation (18–24 Gy in 12 fractions over 2 weeks) and intrathecal (IT) chemotherapy containing methotrexate, cytarabine and hydrocortisone given early in the consolidation phase; IT therapy is continued in the consolidation and maintenance phases; CNS

prophylaxis reduces the rate of CNS relapse from 30 to 75 percent.

3. *Consolidation therapy* to reduce tumor burden further and reduce risk of relapse and development of drug-resistant cells; consists of alternating cycles of induction agents and other cytotoxics; usually includes one or two 'intensification' phases; combinations of methotrexate at high dose, cytarabine, etoposide, *m*-amsacrine, mitoxantrone (mitozantrone) and idarubicin are used.
4. *Maintenance therapy* is necessary for all patients who do not proceed to a stem cell transplant; daily 6-MP and weekly methotrexate for two to three years plus cyclical administration of IV vincristine and IT methotrexate.
5. *Allogeneic stem cell transplantation:* An option for adults <50 with a compatible sibling; leukemia-free survival is superior after first remission allograft in patients with high risk disease (40% *vs.* <10% for Ph+ ALL); treatment-related mortality up to 30 percent; in low risk patients SCT should be reserved for second CR. Matched unrelated donor transplant: an option in younger patients (<40) with very high risk disease (Ph/BCR-ABL positive ALL) but has up to 48 percent treatment-related mortality (Fig. 5.7).

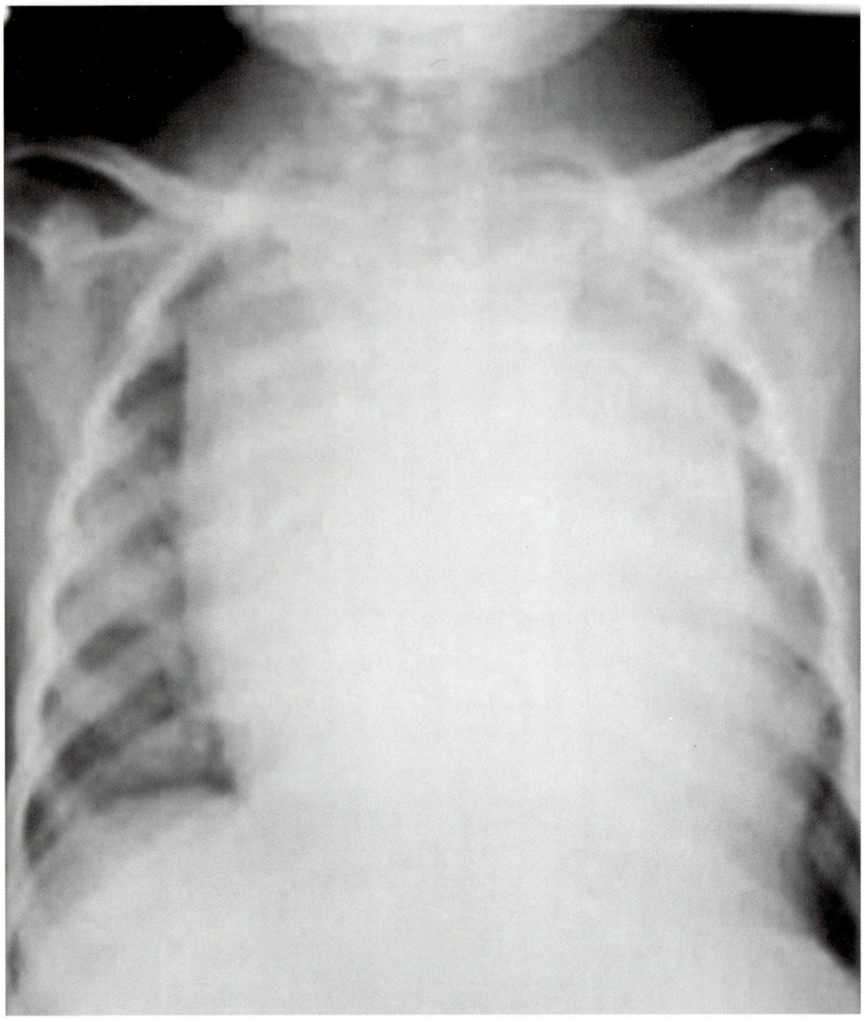

Fig. 5.7: X-ray chest showing marked mediastinal widening in a patient of T-ALL

Prognosis

- Overall ~75 percent of adults with ALL achieve a CR with a modern regimen and good supportive care. In contrast to the high cure rate in childhood ALL, leukemia free survival in adult ALL in general is <30 percent at 5 years (patients > 50 years 10–20%)
- Leukemia-free survival (LFS) after chemotherapy in patients with very high risk Ph/BCR-ABL+ ALL is <10 percent; hence the latter should have an allograft in CR1 if possible.

Criteria for Complete Response to Therapy in Acute Leukemia

- This is defined as less than five percent blasts in the bone marrow
- Evidence of regeneration in the bone marrow by evidence of an acceptable level of cellularity (>20% bone marrow biopsy)
- Restoration of normal hematopoiesis as reflected by peripheral blood values of at least 1500 neutrophils/mm^3 and 1 lac/mm^3 platelets
- No circulating blasts in peripheral blood (in the absence of growth factor use)
- No evidence of extramedullary disease

The above criteria must be sustained for a period of at least four week

At the time of diagnosis 10^{12} cell remain (Leukemic cells) in the body. Standard chemotherapy results in 90 to 99 percent reduction in the total amount of tumor cells. In a state of minimum residual disease (MRD), leukemia burden is 10 billion cells. MRD is best detected by RT PCR assay where total number of cells analyzed is one million and limit of sensitivity of < 0.0001.

ACUTE MYELOID LEUKEMIA (AML)

Acute myeloid leukemia is diagnosed by presence of at least 20 percent myeloblasts in the bone marrow nucleated cells. The only exception is AML M3 which is characterized by presence of abnormal promyelocytes in the blood and bone marrow. According to the FAB classification, AML may be of 8 types as given below:

1. M0— Undifferentiated/minimally differentiated AML (Figs 5.8 and 5.19)

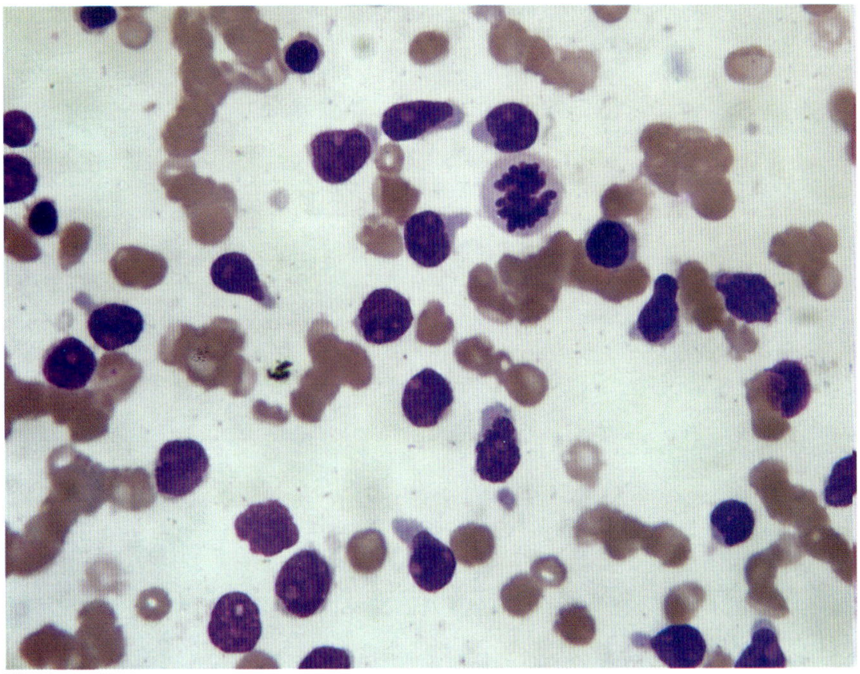

Fig. 5.8: M0–undifferentiated /minimally differentiated AML showing large nucleus with nucleoli and deep blue cytoplasm

2. M1— AML without maturation
3. M2— AML with maturation (Fig. 5.9)
4. M3— Acute promyelocytic leukemia (Fig. 5.10)

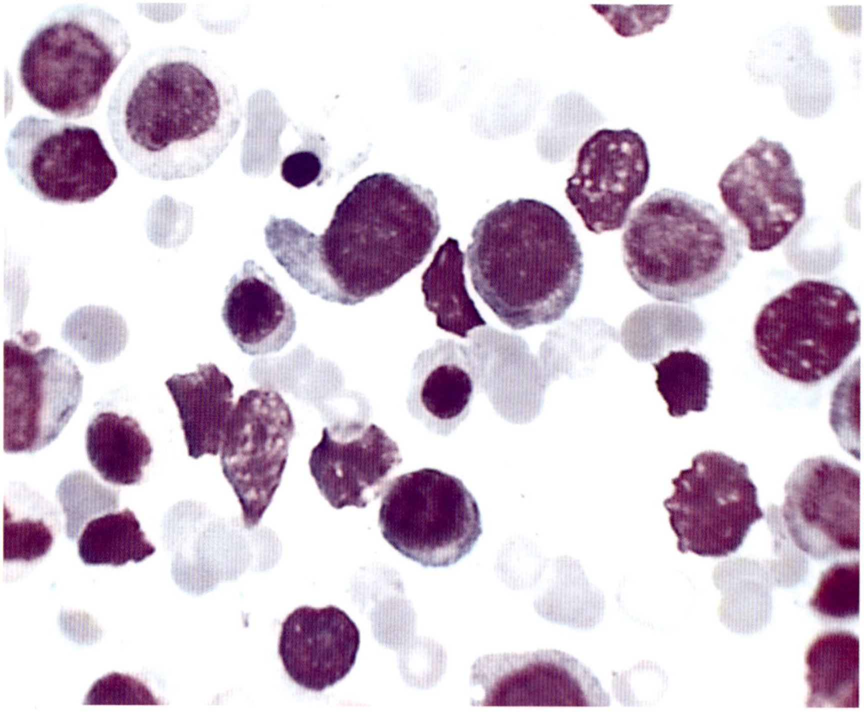

Fig. 5.9: M2—AML with maturation showing large blasts with large nucleus with nucleoli amidst maturing myeloid precursors like myelocytes

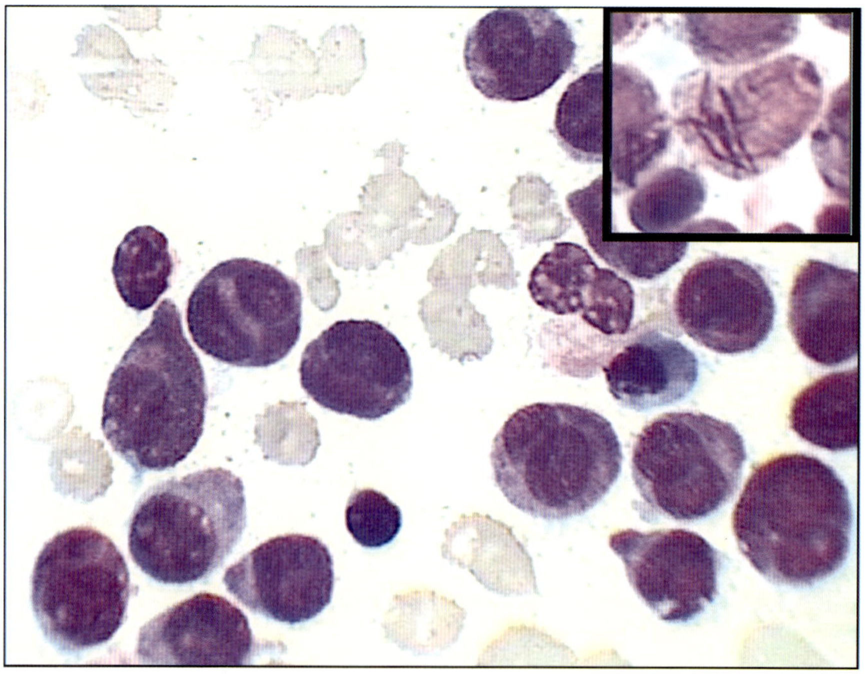

Fig. 5.10: M3—Acute promyelocytic leukemia showing blasts and atypical promyelocytes with bilobed nuclei and prominent granules

5. M4— Acute myelomonocytic leukemia (Fig. 5.11)
6. M5— Acute monoblastic/monocytic leukemia (Fig. 5.12)

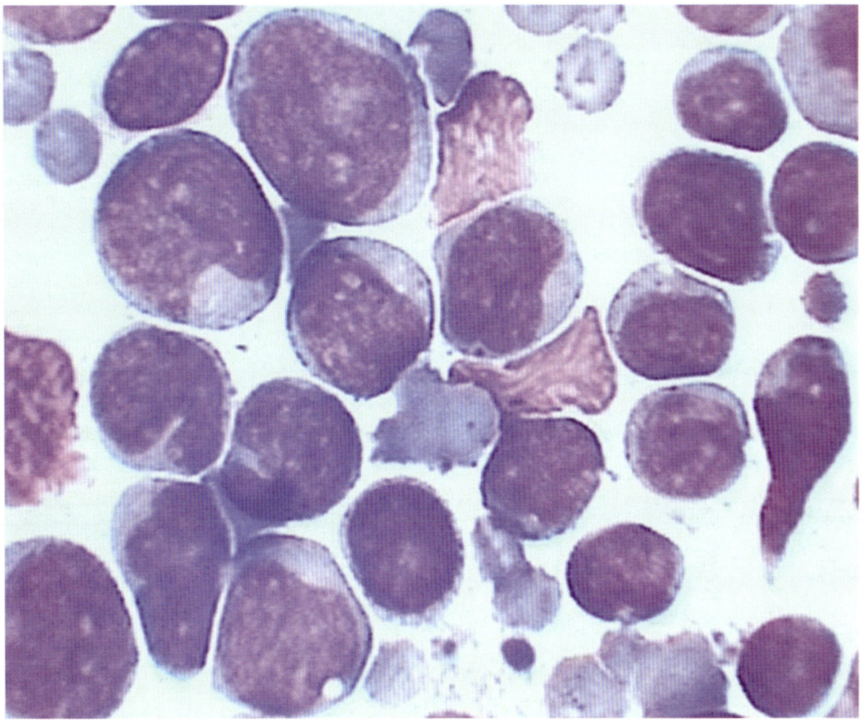

Fig. 5.11: M4—Acute myelomonocytic leukemia showing cellular bone marrow with monoblasts having moderate to large amount of blue cytoplasm and myeloblasts with scant blue cytoplasm

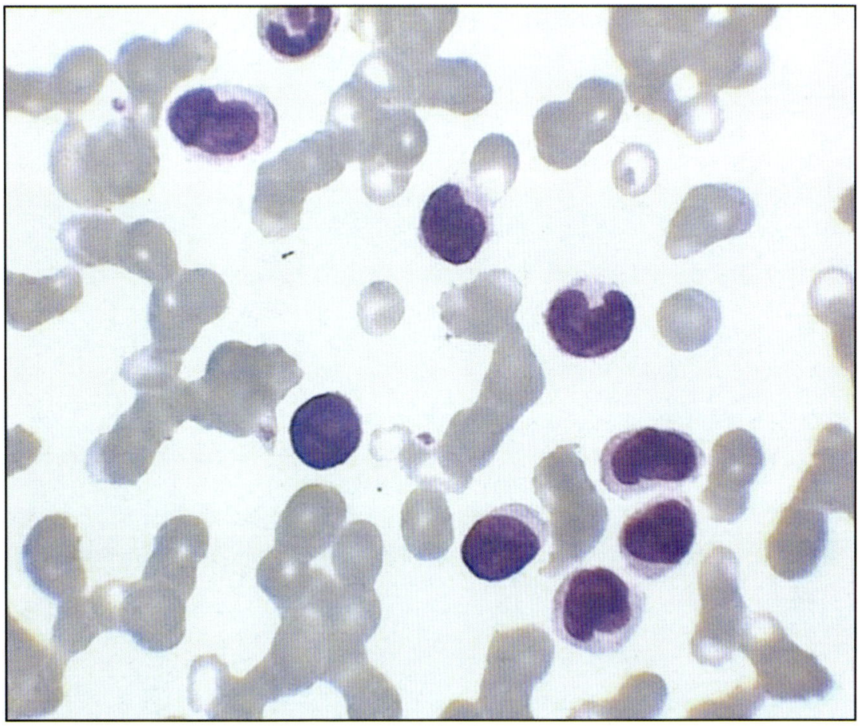

Fig. 5.12: M5—Acute monoblastic/monocytic leukemia showing large blasts and promonocytes

7. M6— AML with erythroid differentiation (Fig. 5.13)
8. M7— Acute megakaryoblastic leukemia (Fig. 5.14)

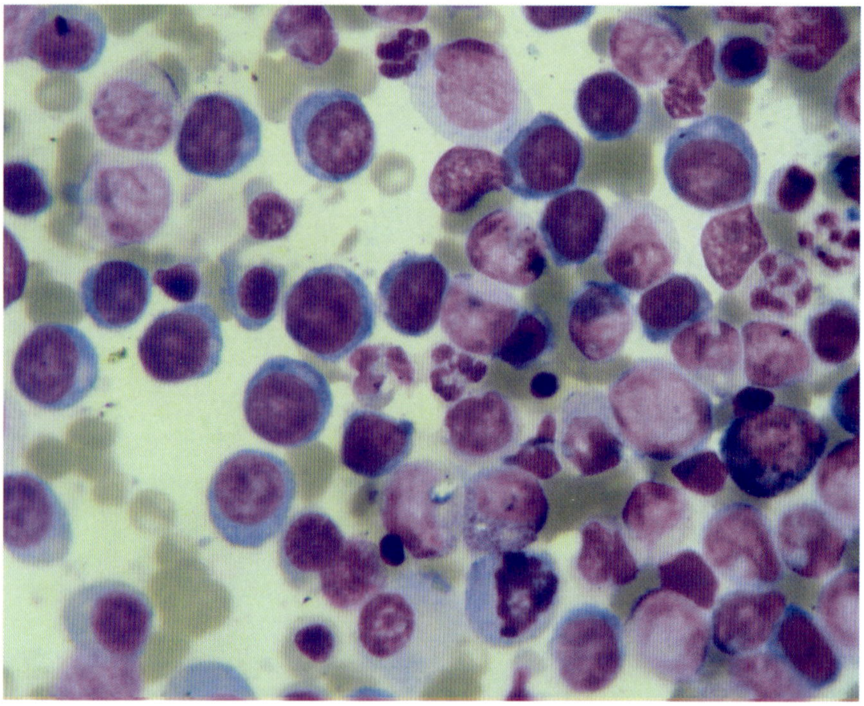

Fig. 5.13: M6—AML with erythroid showing erythroid hyperplasia with dyserythropoiesis, megaloblastosis and gigantoblasts along with nonerythroid blasts

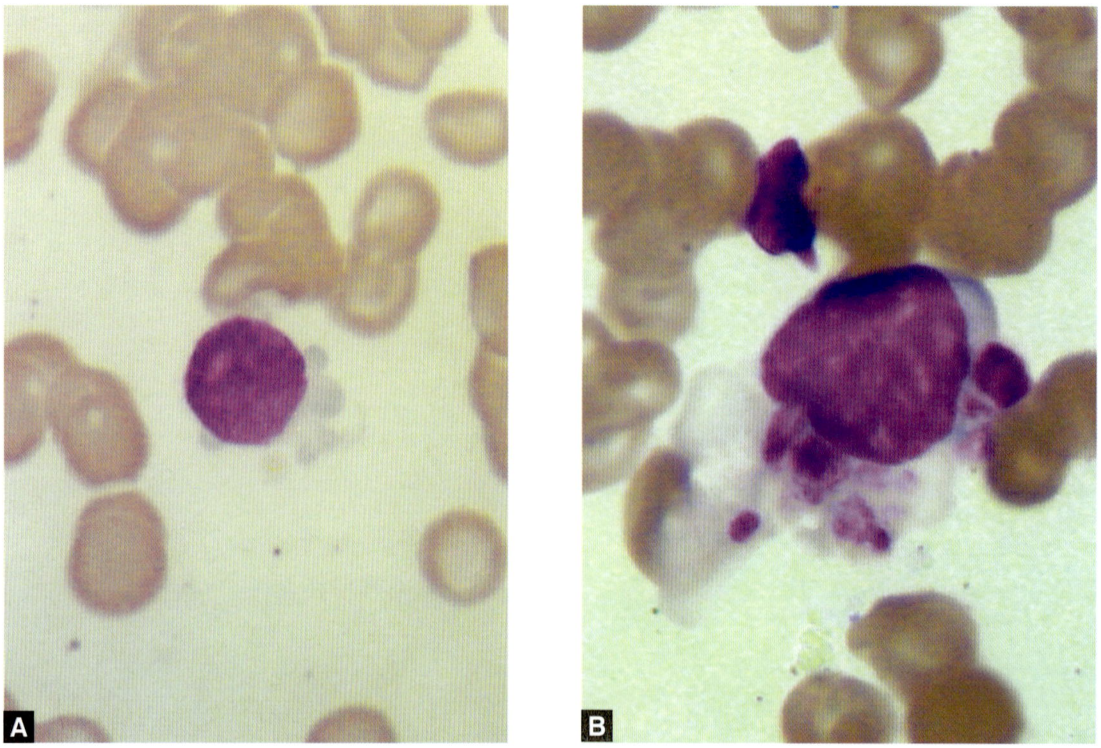

Figs 5.14A and B: Megakaryoblast in AML-M7; (A) Cytoplasmic blebbing; (B) Platelet budding

WHO Categorization of AML

- AML with recurrent cytogenetic abnormalities
- AML with multilineage dysplasia (prior history of myelodysplastic syndrome (MDS) or *de novo*)
- AML, not otherwise categorized (FAB types M0 to M7): therapy or occupation related.

Diagnosis

Blood and Peripheral Smear

The total WBC count may be low, normal or high. Peripheral smear reveals presence of blasts which may have a myeloid morphology. Auer rods or Phi bodies which are collections of primary granules, characteristic of myeloblasts may be seen. Anemia and thrombocytopenia are common.

Bone Marrow

It shows presence of blasts. At least 20 percent of marrow nucleated cells should be blasts or blast equivalent (promonocytes and abnormal promyelocytes in AML M3 are blast equivalents).

Cytochemistry

Sudan black and myeloperoxidase: Myeloblasts are positive for Sudan black (Fig. 5.15) and myeloperoxidase (Fig. 5.16). Promyelocytes are strongly positive:

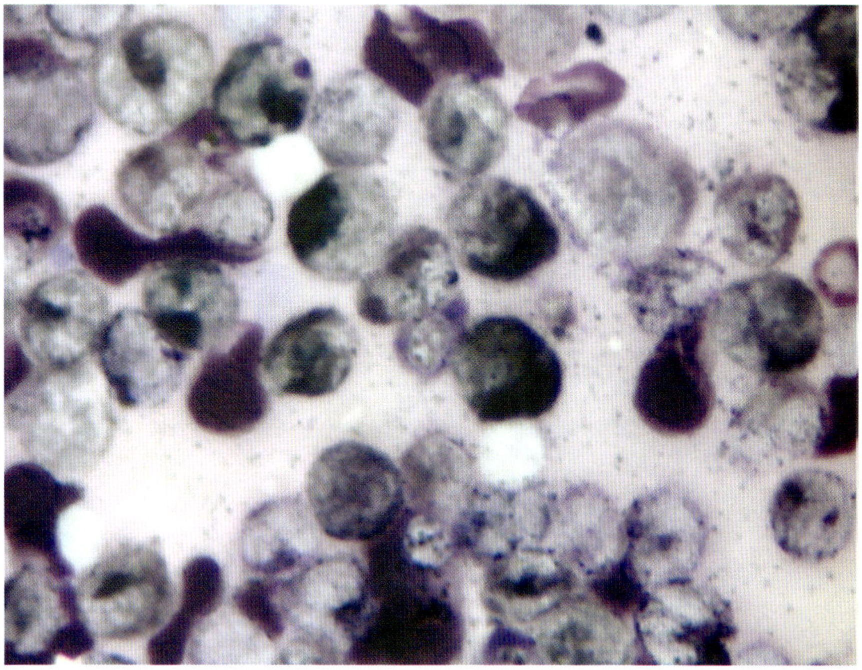

Fig. 5.15: Sudan black (SB) stain showing black granules on blasts

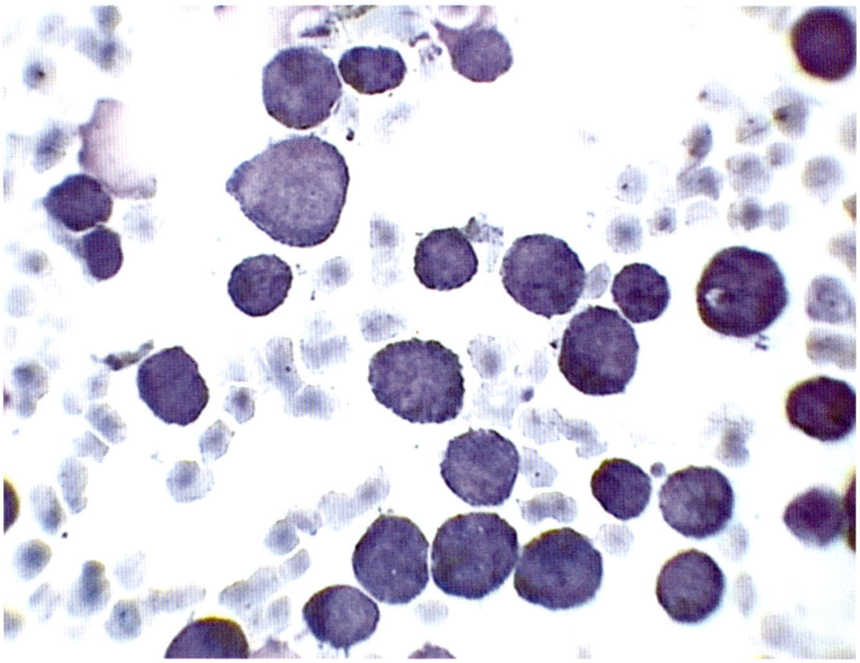

Fig. 5.16: Myeloperoxidase stain (MPO) positivity showing blue granules in blasts

- *Nonspecific Esterase (NSE):* Monoblasts, monocytes are positive for NSE (Fig. 5.17)
- *Dual esterase:* This consists of nonspecific esterase, specific for monocytoid cells (Rust granules) and chloroacetate esterase specific for myeloblasts (Blue granules) (Fig. 5.18). Thus, both esterases are positive in AML-M4 whereas only chloroacetate is positive in M2 and only nonspecific esterase in M5.

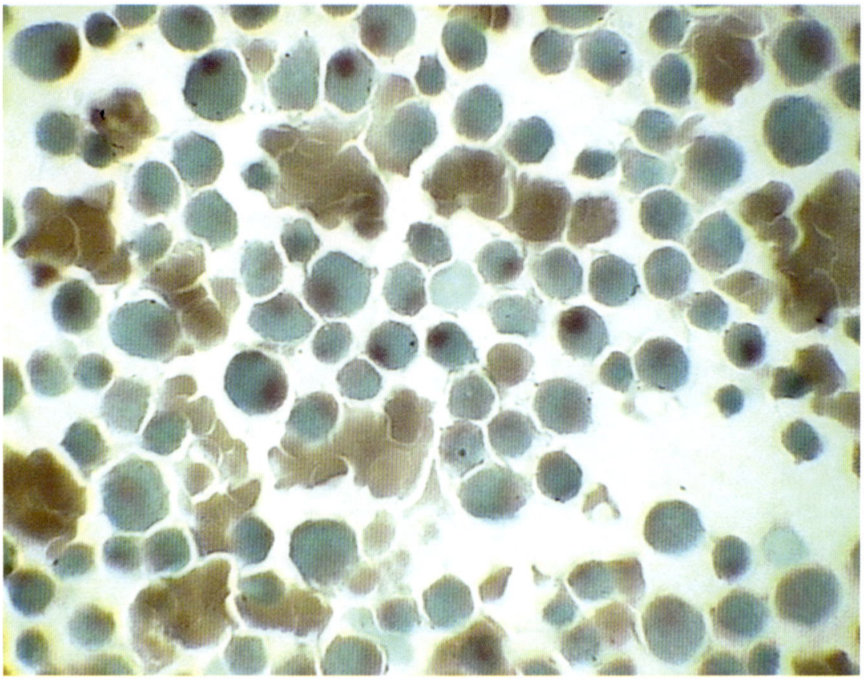

Fig. 5.17: Nonspecific esterase (NSE) showing rust color granules in a monoblasts

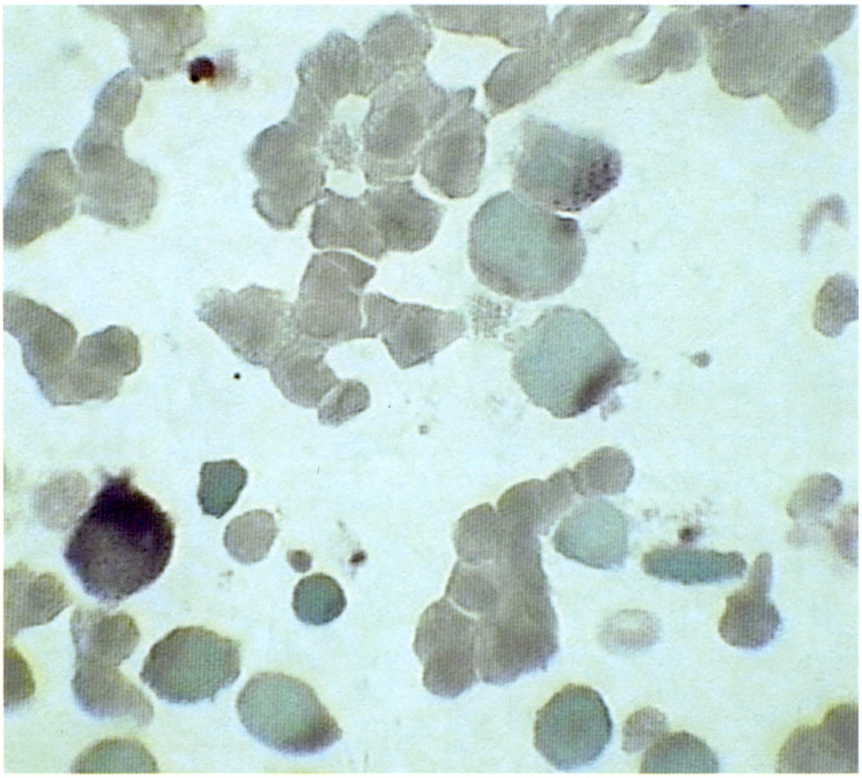

Fig. 5.18: Dual esterase stain showing blasts with chloroacetate esterase positivity (blue granules) as well as nonspecific esterase positivity (Rust colored granules) from a patient with AML M4

Immunophenotyping in Acute Leukemia

This may help in diagnosis sometimes when cytochemistry is not helpful as in M0, M7 or biphenotypic leukemia (Table 5.1).

Electron Microscopy

Ultrastructural study may be useful in diagnosis in some cases especially AML M0 (Fig. 5.19), AML M7 and biphenotypic leukemia.

Table 5.1: Suggested panel of diagnostic antibodies

	Primary panel	*Supplementary panel*
B-Lymphoid	CD19; CD10; cy CD22	Cy μ, SmIg
T-lymphoid	CD7; CD2; cyCD 3	CD5; CD1; CD4; CD8
Myeloid	CD13; CD33; anti-MPO	CD41; CD61; anti-glycophorin
Nonlineage related	TdT	

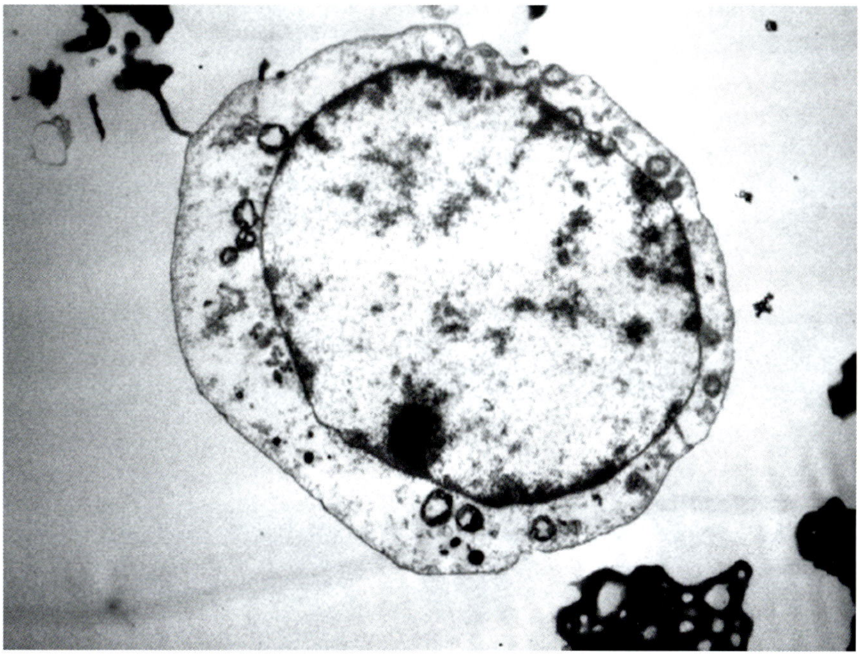

Fig. 5.19: AML M0 (EM=16000 m): Ultrastructural myeloid blast showing cytoplasmic granules which are MPO positive

BIPHENOTYPIC LEUKEMIA

Biphenotypic or Mixed Lineage Acute Leukemias

They account for five percent of cases and are characterized by the coexpression of a constellation of myeloid and lymphoid antigen in the blasts cells (Table 5.2).

Interpretation: Biphenotyping leukemia is defined when scores for the myeloid and one of the lymphoid lineages are greater than 2 points. Each marker scores the corresponding point. Cases of ALL or AML with expression of myeloid or lymphoid markers respectively but with scores less than 2.5 point have been described as myeloid antigen+ ALL and lymphoid antigen + AML respectively. In contrast to biphenotypic acute leukaemia, they do not seem to be cytogenetically or prognostically different from ALL or AML with no aberrant antigen expression.

Most specific markers score 2, for example CD3 for the T-lymphoid lineage , Cd79a, Ig and CD22 for the B-lymphoid lineage and anti-MPO for the myeloid lineage. EM also helps in diagnosis.

AML WITH MULTILINEAGE DYSPLASIA

Multilineage dysplasia: There is presence of at least 50 percent dysplastic cells in two or more cell lines. It is typically but not exclusively seen in older patients. Its complete remission rate is lower.

Chromosomal abnormalities: Gain or loss of chromosomal material is more common, e.g. –5, –7, 7q–, +8, +9, +11,17p–, 20q–, and translocations are less common e.g.: t(3;21), t(3;5), t(1:7), and t(2;11).

ACUTE MYELOBLASTIC LEUKEMIA/MYELODYSPLASTIC SYNDROME: OCCUPATION RELATED OR THERAPY RELATED

This occurs secondary to toxic exposure like benzene and related petrochemicals, may be therapy related, e.g. secondary to alkylating agents or secondary to therapy with topoisomerase II inhibitors.

Criteria for Complete Response to Therapy in Acute Leukemia

- This is defined as less than five percent blasts in the bone marrow
- Evidence of regeneration in the bone marrow by evidence of an acceptable level of cellularity (>20% bone marrow biopsy)
- Restoration of normal hematopoiesis as reflected by peripheral blood values of at least 1500 neutrophils/cumm and 1 lac/cumm platelets

Table 5.2: Scoring system for the diagnosis of biphenotypic leukemia

Score	*B-Lymphoid*	*T-Lymphoid*	*Myeloid*
2	CD 79a	CD 3	Anti MPO
	Cyt CD 22	Anti- TCR $\alpha\beta$	
	Cyt IgM	Anti- TCR $\gamma\delta$	
1	CD 19	CD 2	CD 117
	CD 20	CD 5	CD 13
	CD 10	CD 8	CD 33
		CD 10	CD 65
0.5	TdT	TdT	CD 14
	CD 24	CD 7	CD 15
			CD 68

MPO: Myeloperoxidase; TCR: T-cell receptor; TdT: Terminal deoxynucleotidyl transferase

- No circulating blasts in peripheral blood (in the absence of growth factor use)
- No evidence of extramedullary disease.

The above criteria must be sustained for a period of at least four weeks.

Clinical Features

Acute myeloid leukemia (AML) is primarily an adult disease with a median age at presentation of 60 years and an increasing incidence with advanced age:

- Acute presentation usual; often critically ill due to effects of bone marrow failure
- *Symptoms of anemia:* Weakness, lethargy, breathlessness, lightheadedness and palpitations
- *Infection:* Particularly chest, mouth, perianal, skin (*Staphylococcus*, *Pseudomonas*, HSV, *Candida and harpes zoster*). (Figs 5.20 and 5.21)

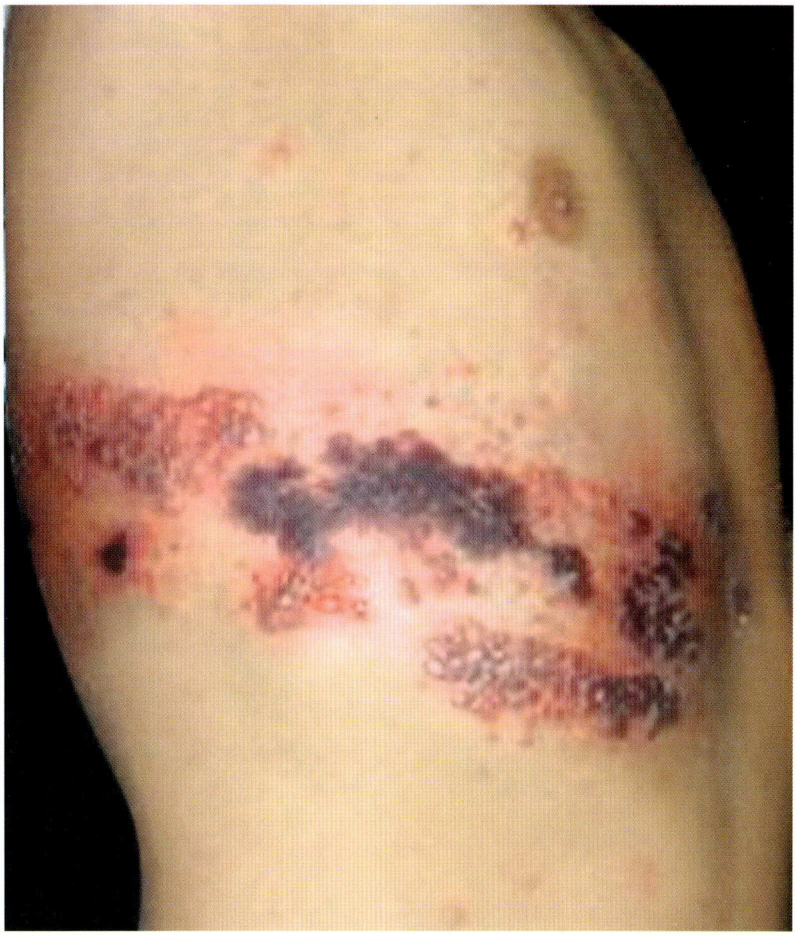

Fig. 5.20: Herpes zoster in a patient with ALL during chemotherapy

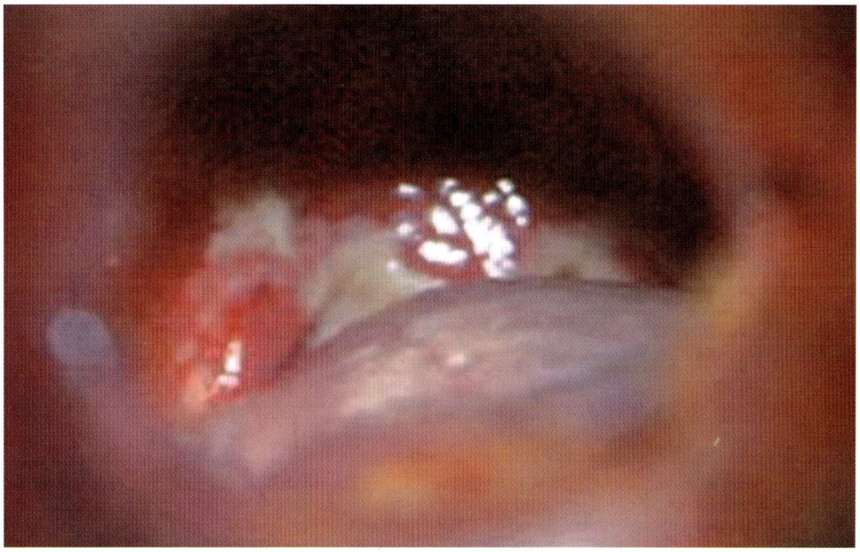

Fig. 5.21: Oral candidiasis in a patient with neutropenia following chemotherapy

- *Hemorrhage (especially M3 due to DIC):* Purpura, menorrhagia and epistaxis, bleeding gums, rectal, retina.
- Gum hypertrophy and skin infiltration (M4, M5) (Figs 5.22 and 5.23)

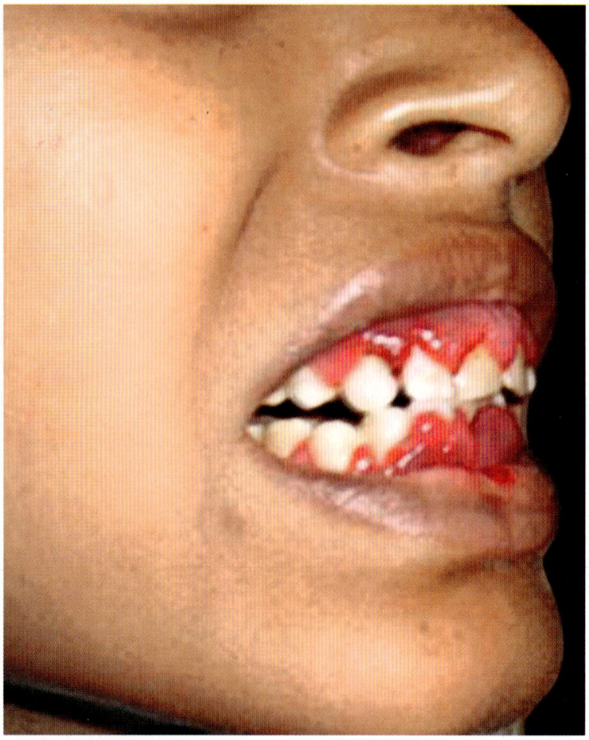

Fig. 5.22: Gum hypertrophy in a patient of acute monoblastic leukemia

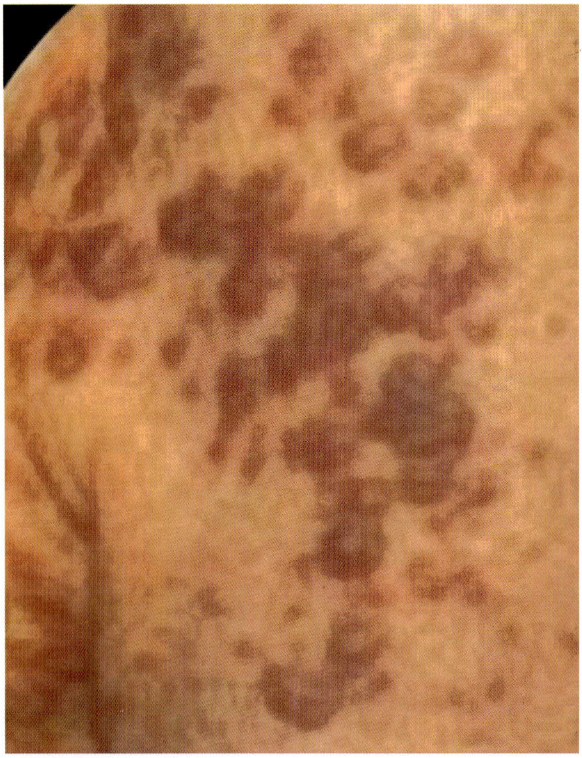

Fig. 5.23: Leukemia cutis in a patient of acute myeloid leukemia (FAB-M4)

- Signs of leukostasis, e.g. hypoxia, retinal hemorrhage, confusion or diffuse pulmonary shadowing (Fig. 5.24)
- Hepatomegaly occurs in 20 percent, splenomegaly in 24 percent; the latter should raise the question of transformed CML; lymphadenopathy is infrequent (17%)
- CNS involvement at presentation is rare in adults with AML
- Skin involvement (leukemia cutis) occurs in approximately 10 percent of patients and usually presents as violaceous, raised, nontender plaques or nodules, which on biopsy are found to be infiltrated with myeloblasts. More common in monocytic leukemic subtypes
- Sweet syndrome (acute neutrophilic dermatosis) is a cutaneous paraneoplastic syndrome that is associated with AML (more common in the monocytic leukemias) and other hematologic disorders. It is characterized by fever and tender red plaques and nodules usually on the extremities. Sweet syndrome may precede the diagnosis of AML by several months. The histologic finding in Sweet syndrome consists of a dense infiltrate primarily composed of mature neutrophils

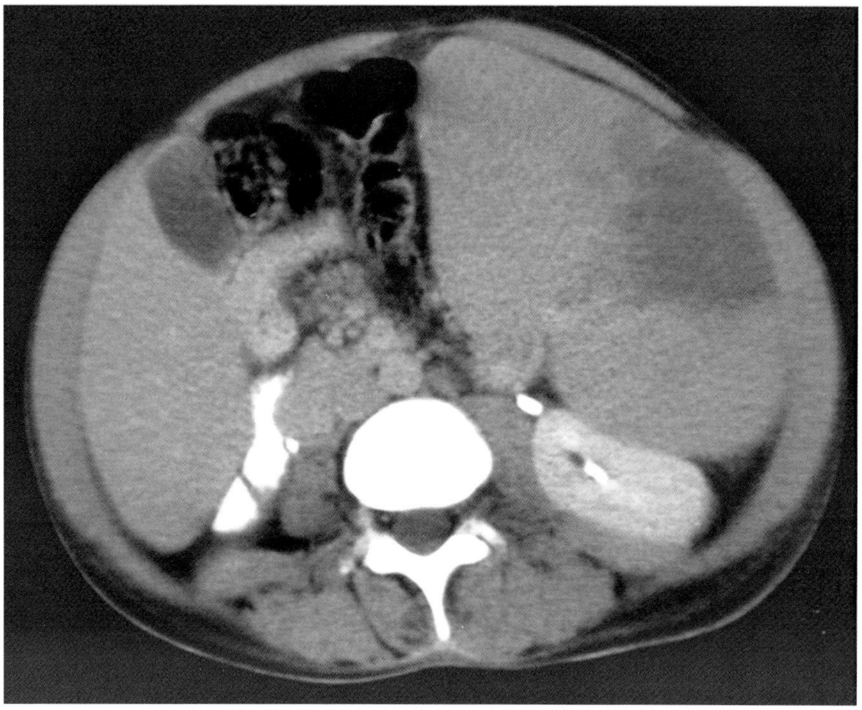

Fig. 5.24: CT abdomen showing splenic infarction in a patient with leukemia with leukocytosis

- Myeloid granulocytic sarcomas (chloromas) are collections of blasts in extramedullary sites, which may present as isolated subcutaneous masses and may be confused with a primary or metastatic carcinoma. The term *chloromas* is derived from the greenish appearance on sectioning, which is secondary to the presence of myeloperoxidase (MPO) granules in the myeloblasts. Myeloid sarcomas may precede the development of AML and are more common in the undifferentiated and minimally differentiated AML subtypes. Chloromas are generally associated with poor prognosis (Fig. 5.25).

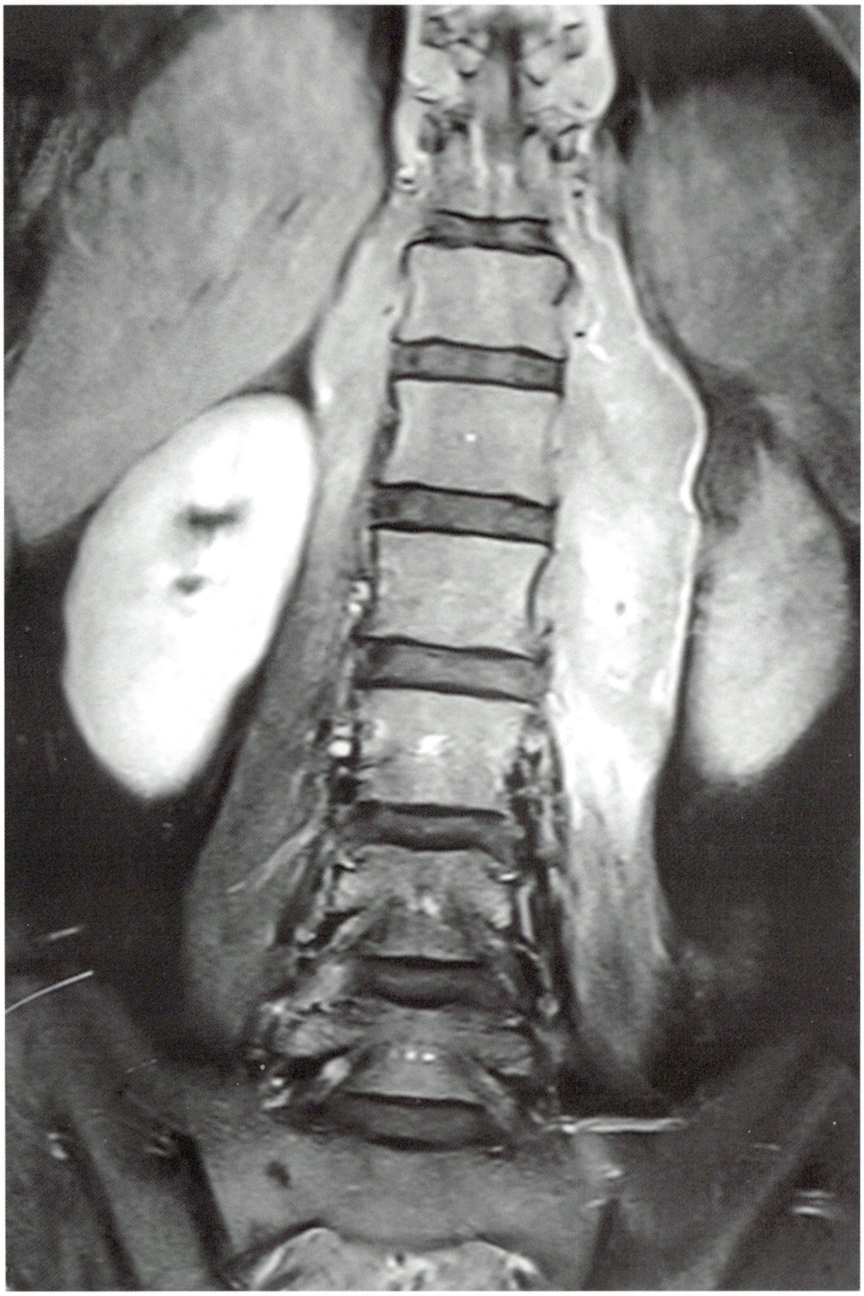

Fig. 5.25: Granulocytic sarcoma at paravertebral area in a patient of AML-M2

Prognostic Factors

The most important prognostic factors predicting for achievement of remission and for subsequent relapse are:

- Advancing patient age; <50 favorable; >60 unfavorable
- Presenting leukocyte count; <25 × 10^9/L favorable; >100 × 10^9/L unfavorable
- History of antecedent MDS or leukemogenic therapy, unfavorable
- Presence of specific cytogenetic abnormalities
- FAB subtype: M3, M4Eo favorable; M0, M7 unfavorable
- Failure to achieve CR with first cycle of induction therapy predicts for relapse.

Treatment

- Treatment protocols are age related; patients >60 only tolerate less intensive treatments and very rarely transplantation
- Supportive treatment alone is a valid treatment option in the >75 age group or if there are coexistent serious general medical problems.
- For patients <60 years—four to five courses of intensive combination chemotherapy initially including daunorubicin or another anthracycline and cytosine arabinoside each lasting five to ten days with a two to three week period of profound myelosuppression
- The use of all-*trans*-retinoic acid (ATRA) with initial therapy reduces the risk of DIC. After this the prognosis is good. ATRA induces differentiation of the abnormal clone by overcoming the molecular block resulting from the t(15;17) translocation. ATRA alone cannot achieve sustained remission but in combination with chemotherapy 70 percent of patients may be cured.

Prognosis

- Seventy to eighty percent of patients aged <60 years will achieve a CR with a modern regimen and good supportive care; more intensive induction and consolidation regimens reduce the risk of relapse
- Relapse risk at five years in patients <60 with favorable risk cytogenetics is 29 to 42 percent; intermediate risk 39 to 60 percent; poor risk 68 to 90 percent
- Fifty to sixty percent of patients aged ≥60 years achieve CR with induction treatment (rate drops with each decade) but relapse occurs in 80 to 90 percent; a higher proportion have poor risk karyotype, previous myelodysplasia and comorbidity; treatment-related morbidity and mortality is high.

CHAPTER 6

Chronic Leukemia

CHAPTER OVERVIEW

- Chronic myeloid leukemia (CML)
- Polycythemia vera
- Essential thrombocythemia
- Chronic lymphocytic leukemia
- Prolymphocytic leukemia (PLL)
- Hairy cell leukemia (HCL)

Chronic leukemias are characterized by accumulation of mature cells. They are characterized by a more insidious and chronic course. Nevertheless, ultimately signs and symptoms of marrow failure set in as these differentiated neoplastic cells are abnormal and often functionally useless and also these chronic leukemias often undergo a blastic transformation, wherein blasts cells start accumulating. They are predominantly of two types: Chronic leukemias may be chronic myeloid leukemia (CML) or chronic lymphocytic leukemia (CLL).

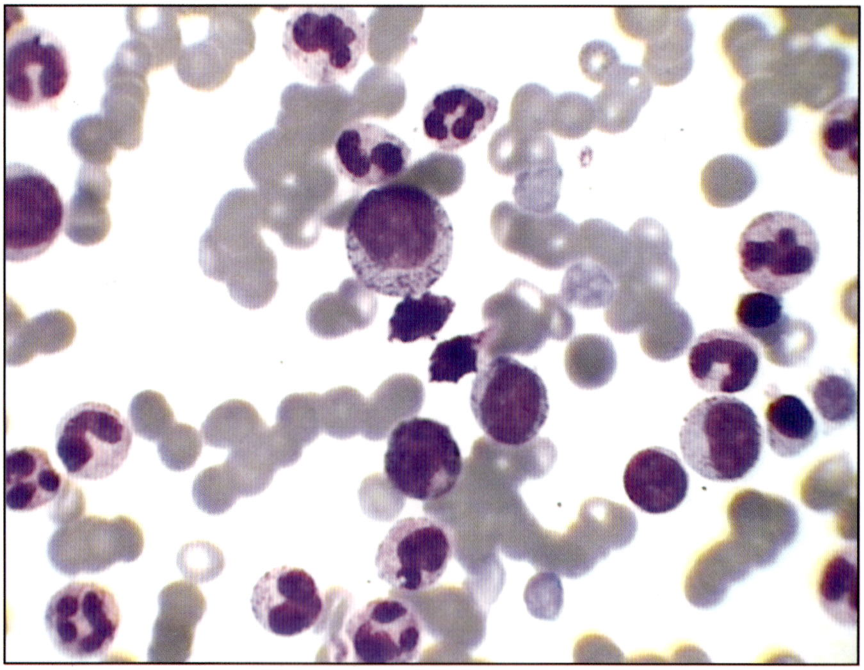

Fig. 6.1: Peripheral smear in CML showing leukocytosis and myeloid precursors along with basophils

CHRONIC MYELOID LEUKEMIA (CML)

This constitutes 15 percent of all leukemias and is a malignant disorder of multipotent stem cells with predominance of mature granulocytes and their precursors accumulating in excess in the marrow and blood (Fig. 6.1).

Special stains: LAP (leukocyte alkaline phosphatase) activity in leukocytes of CML is abnormally low or absent. This helps to differentiate from reactive conditions like leukemoid reactions. In leukemoid reaction, the LAP score is high whereas in CML it is very low (Fig. 6.2).

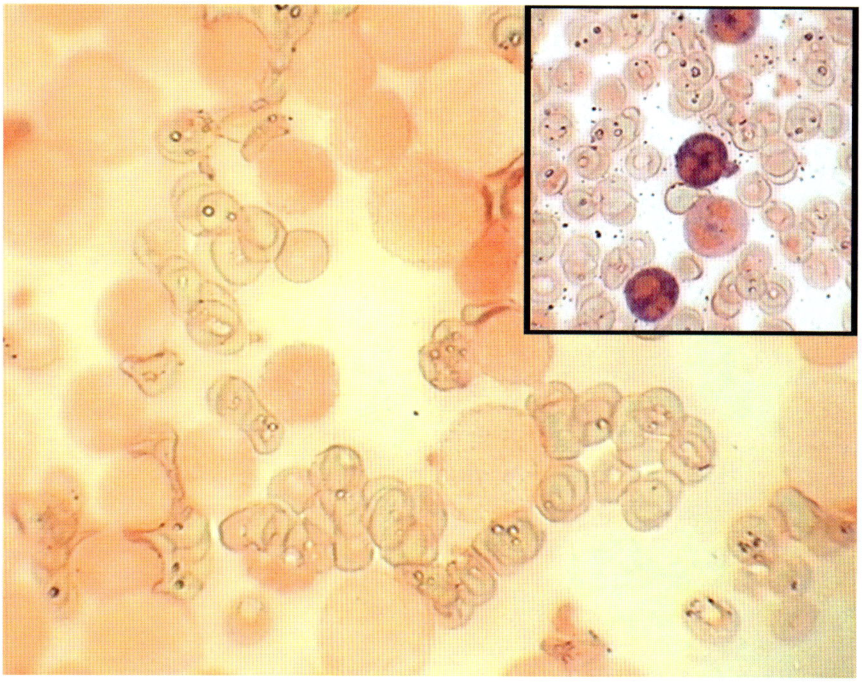

Fig. 6.2: Leukocytes alkaline phosphatase (LAP) showing absent LAP activity with inset showing blue granules (3+) in normal neutrophil

Diagnosis

Blood and peripheral smear: The peripheral blood WBC count of stable CML is typically elevated from 20 x 10^9/l, and is often >100 x10^9/l. Segmented neutrophils, myelocytes, and metamyelocytes predominate, but eosinophilia and basophilia are characteristic findings in CML peripheral smear. Anemia is usually only moderate. Platelet numbers may be normal or elevated (50%) in most of the patients.

Note: Sometimes chronic myeloid leukemia may present for the first time with blast crisis. In such cases, it may be difficult to differentiate from acute leukemia. Presence of associated massive splenomegaly gives a clue to underlying CML. In such cases it is important to search for presence of basophils since their presence suggests underlying CML. This can be confirmed by presence of Philadelphia chromosome/BCR-ABL transcript.

Bone marrow: The bone marrow is hypercellular (100%) with a great increase in the M:E ratio; a left-shifted myeloid series, and increased eosinophils. Megakaryocytes may be normal or elevated and are often smaller than normal.

Phases of Chronic Myeloid Leukemia

1. *Chronic phase:* This is diagnosed when blasts less than 10% in peripheral smear and less than 10% in bone marrow.
2. *Accelerated phase (Fig. 6.3):* criteria?
   - Blasts in peripheral blood — 10-19 percent
   - Persistent increase
   - Peripheral blood basophils — ≥ 20 percent
   - Persistent LBC count platelet count
   - Platelets ≤ 1 lac unrelated to therapy
   - Persistent or increasing spleen size
   - Cytogenetic evolution
3. *Blast crisis (Fig. 6.4):*
   - > 20% blasts in p/s or marrow or both
   - Extramedullary infiltration of leukemic cells (Fig. 6.4)
   - Blasts are lymphoid in 20 percent (TdT+, CD10+, CD19+, CD20+, frequent coexpression of myeloid markers) and myeloid in 70 percent and undifferentiated, erythroid, etc. in 5 to 10 percent.

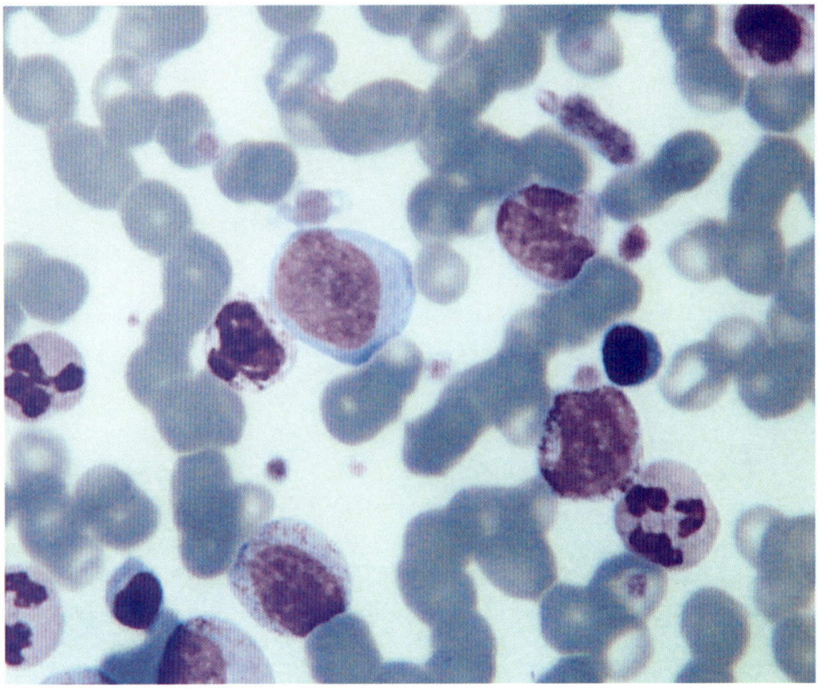

Fig. 6.3: CML (AP) showing blast, basophils and myelocytes

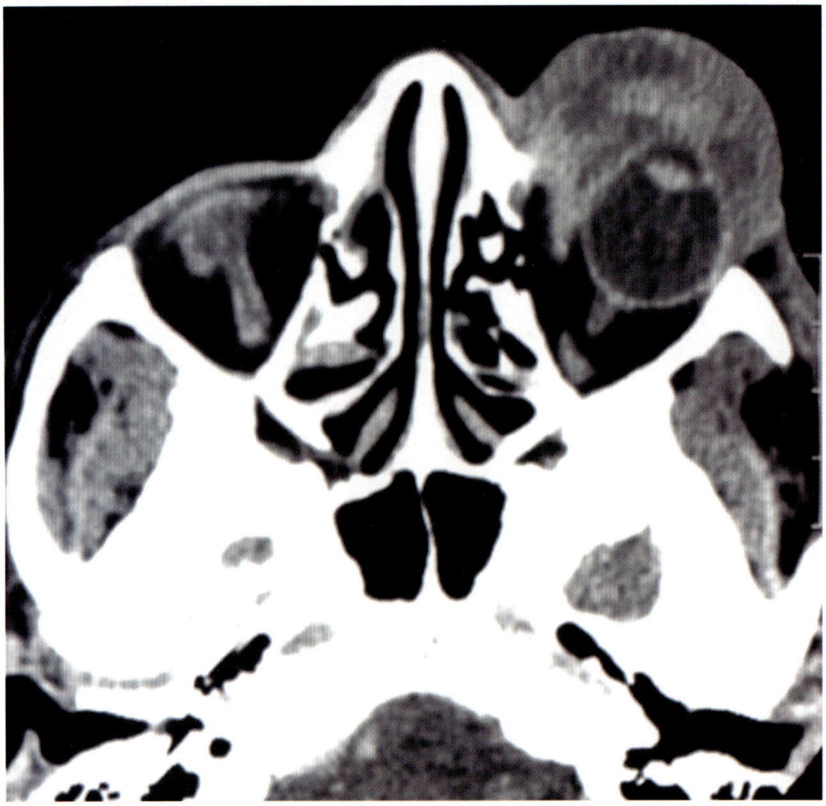

Fig. 6.4: A case CML with blast crisis presented with proptosis of left eye

Sometimes CML may be confused with atypical CML or chronic myelomonocytic leukemia (CMML). These may be differentiated in Table 6.1.

Table 6.1: CML, atypical CML and CMML

Criteria	*CML*	*Atypical CML*	*CMML*
Basophils	> 2%	< 2%	< 2%
Monocytes	< 3%	> 3–10%	> 3–10% (usually >10%)
Granulocyte dysplasia	–	++	+
Immature granulocytes	> 20%	> 10-20%	< 10%
Blasts	< 2%	> 2%	< 2%
BM erythroid cells	Low	Low	Normal

Note

- Atypical CMLs have a male preponderance and present in elderly patients (15–20 years older than patients of CML)
- The TLC in atypical CML is lesser than in CML
- Anemia and thrombocytopenia are more common in atypical CML. These patients usually are symptomatic at presentation
- Bone marrow M:E ratio is less than 10:1 in atypical CML
- Philadelphia chromosome is negative in atypical CML.

Clinical Symptoms and Signs

- Thirty percent asymptomatic at diagnosis; present after routine FBC
- Fatigue, lethargy, weight loss, sweats
- Splenomegaly in >75 percent; may cause (L) hypochondrial pain, satiety and sensation of abdominal fullness (Fig. 6.5)
- Gout, bruising/bleeding, splenic infarction and occasionally priapism
- Signs include moderate to large splenomegaly (40% >10 cm), hepatomegaly (2%), lymphadenopathy unusual
- Occasional signs of leukostasis at presentation.

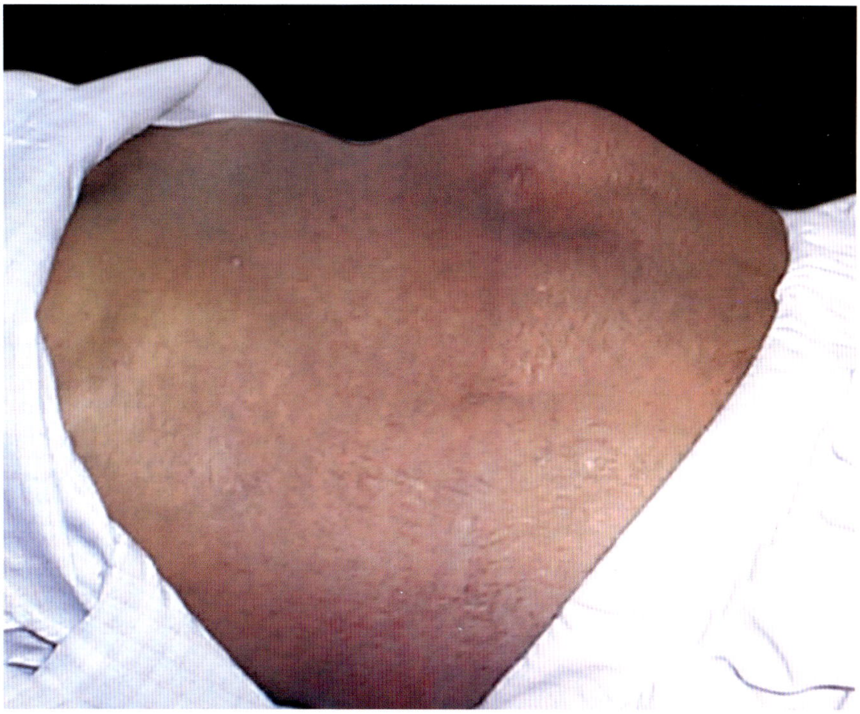

Fig. 6.5: A patient of CML presented with massive splenomegaly

Treatment

- Tyrosine kinase inhibitor—Imatinib mesylate is standard of care in a patient of chronic phase. Complete cytogenetic response of 85 percent at five years.
- Second generation TKI (Dasatinib, Nilotinib) have become available, more potent than imatinib, to be used in patients showing poor response to imatinib or are intolerant.
- Allogenic stem cell transplant is only curative option as of now but with excellent outcome being achieved with imatinib, it is not recommended in a chronic phase patient. In accelerated phase or blast crisis patients, it remains standard of care.

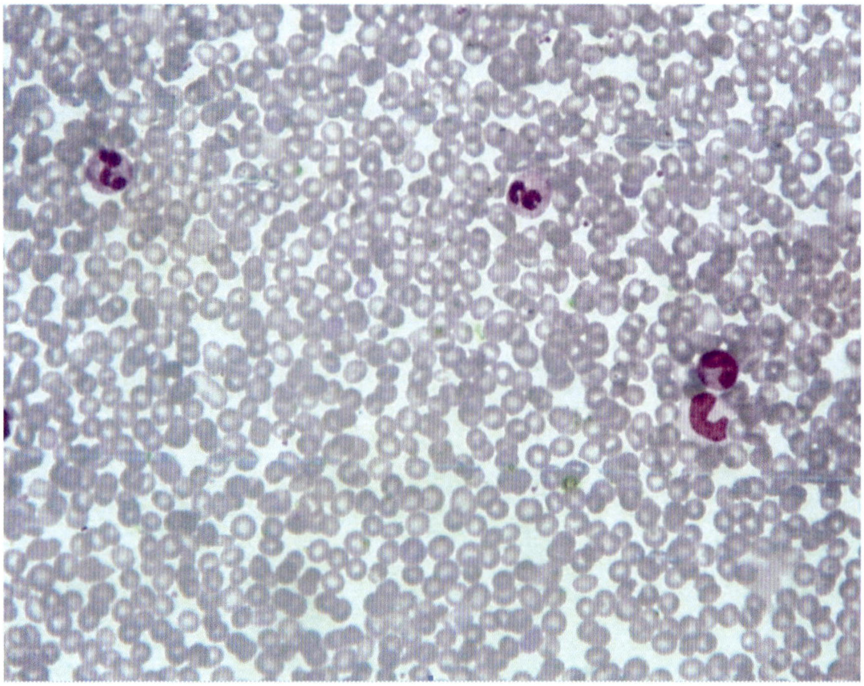

Fig. 6.6: Polycythemia vera—peripheral smear showing red cell crowding

POLYCYTHEMIA VERA (FIGS 6.6 AND 6.7)

Polycythemia vera is a myeloproliferative neoplasm characterized by increased red cell production. Diagnosis requires exclusion of secondary causes of polycythemia and other MPNs. More than 90 percent cases have somatic gain of function mutation of Janus 2 kinase gene (JAK2 V617F) or other functionally similar mutation.

WHO criteria for polycythemia vera: Diagnosis requires the presence of both major and one minor criterion or the presence of the first major criterion together with two minor criteria.

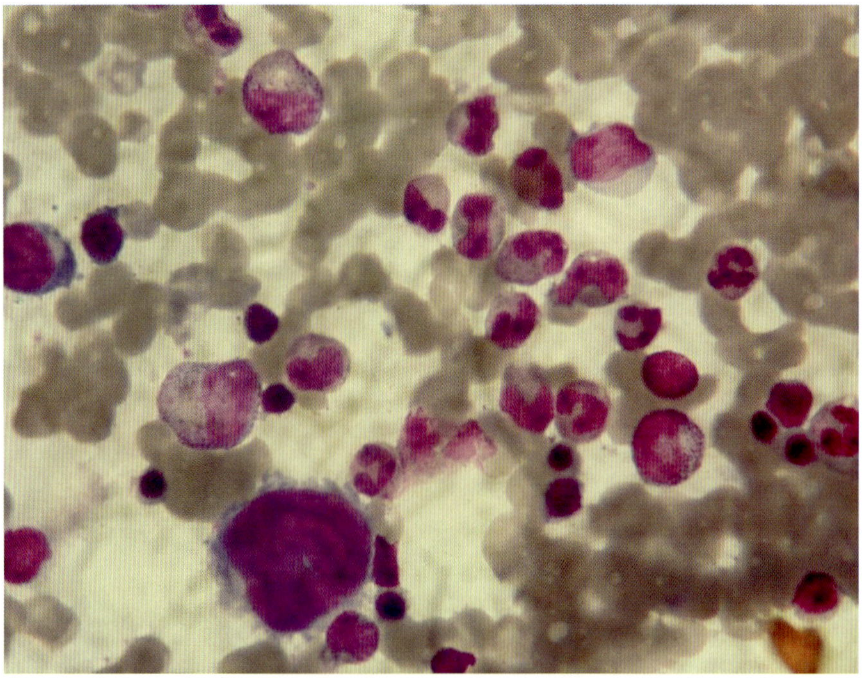

Fig. 6.7: Polycythemia vera—bone marrow showing trilineage proliferation

Major Criteria

- Hemoglobin >18.5 g/dl in men, 16.5 g/dl in women or other evidence of increased red cell volume*.
- Presence of JAK2 V617F or other functionally similar mutation such as JAK2 exon 12 mutation.

Minor Criteria

- Bone marrow biopsy showing hypercellularity for age with trilineage growth (panmyelosis) with prominent erythroid, granulocytic and megakaryocytic proliferation (Fig. 6.7)
- Serum erythropoietin level below the reference range for normal
- Endogenous erythroid colony formation *in vitro*.

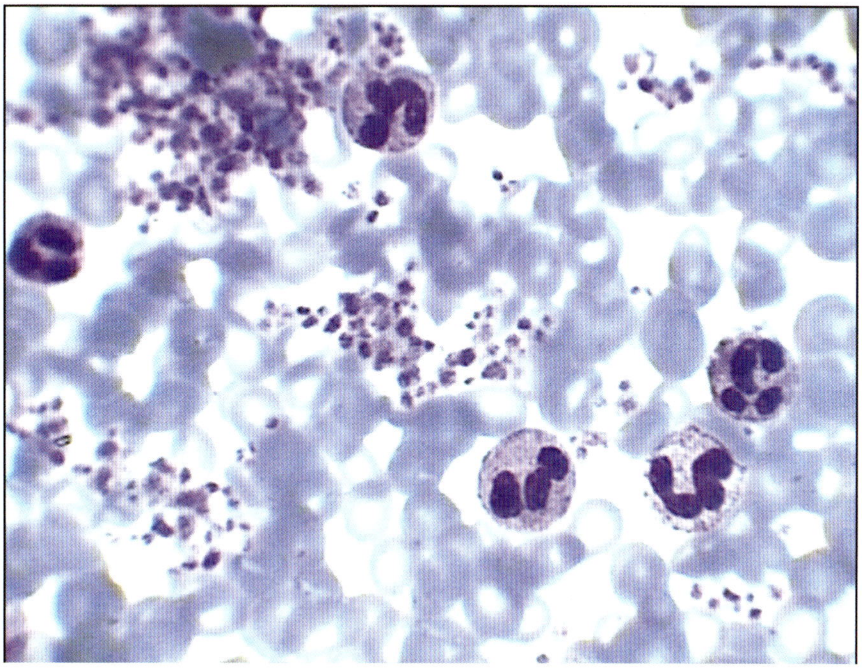

Fig. 6.8: Essential thrombocythemia—peripheral smear showing thrombocytosis

ESSENTIAL THROMBOCYTHEMIA (FIGS 6.8 AND 6.9)

Essential thrombocythemia is a myeloproliferative neoplasm involving primarily the megakaryocytic lineage characterized by persistent thrombocytosis and increased number of large mature megakaryocytes in the bone marrow.

WHO criteria for essential thrombocythemia: Diagnosis requires meeting all four criteria.

- Sustained platelet count $\geq 450 \times 10^9/l$ (Fig. 6.8)
- Bone marrow biopsy showing proliferation mainly of the megakaryocytic lineage with increased numbers of enlarged, mature megakaryocytes (Fig. 6.9). No significant increase or

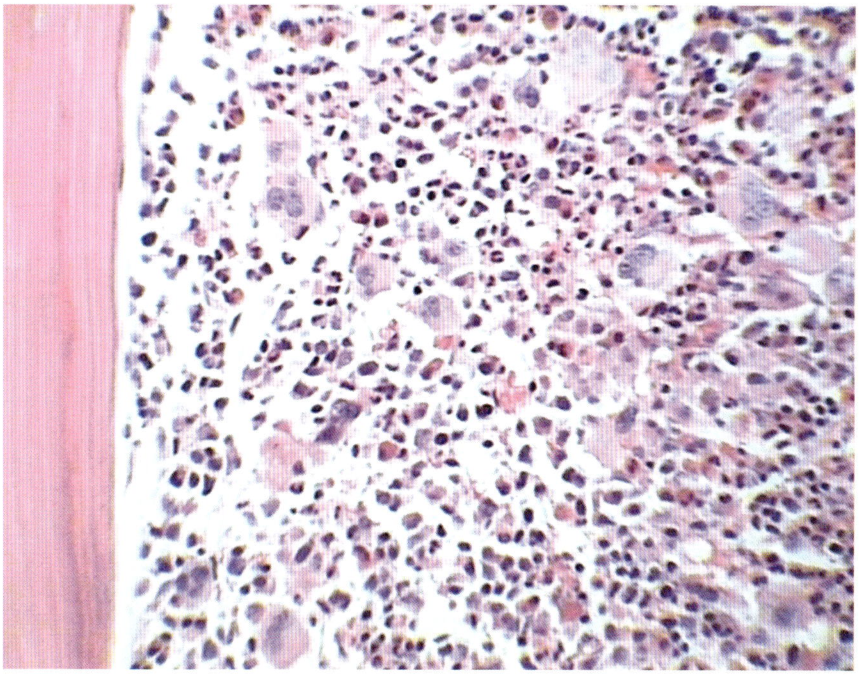

Fig. 6.9: Essential thrombocythemia—bone marrow biopsy showing megakaryocyte clustering

*Hb or Hct >99th percentile of the range for age, sex, altitude of residence or Hb >17 g/dl in men, 15 g/dl in women if associated with a documented and sustained increase of at least 2 g/dl from an individual's baseline value that cannot be attributed to correction of iron deficiency, or elevated red cell mass >25 percent above mean normal predicted value

left shift of neutrophil granulpoiesis or erythropoiesis.
- Not meeting WHO criteria for polycythemia vera, primary myelofibrosis, BCR ABL1 positive chronic myelogenous leukemia or myelodysplastic syndrome or other myeloid neoplasm.
- Demonstration of JAK2 V617F or other clonal marker or in the absence of JAK2 V617F, no evidence for reactive thrombocytosis.

CHRONIC LYMPHOCYTIC LEUKEMIA (CLL) (FIGS 6.10 TO 6.12)

CLL is a proliferation of mature appearing, but functionally incompetent lymphocytes, in the marrow, peripheral blood, and various organs. The most characteristic feature of CLL is a peripheral blood absolute lymphocytosis (>5.0 × 10^9/L with typical immunophenotype).

Diagnosis

Blood and peripheral smear: The total count is raised with absolute lymphocytosis. CLL lymphocytes are generally smaller than normal and appear to be more fragile. Large number of "smudge" cells are seen (ruptured lymphocytes/basket cells) (Fig. 6.10). Often, prolymphocytes may also be seen. If they are less than 15 percent, it is termed CLL. If they are 15 to 55 percent, it is termed as CLL/PLL syndrome, which behaves as CLL, but if they are more than 55 percent diagnosis of prolymphocytic leukemia (PLL) is made which behaves worse than CLL.

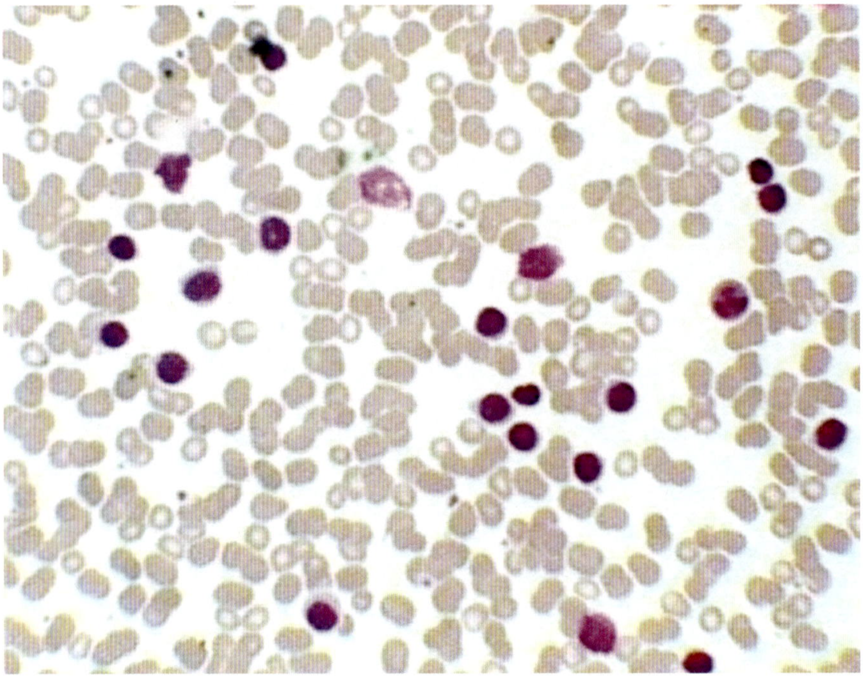

Fig. 6.10: Chronic lymphocytic leukemia—Peripheral smear showing leukocytosis with mature lymophcytes and degenerated basket cells

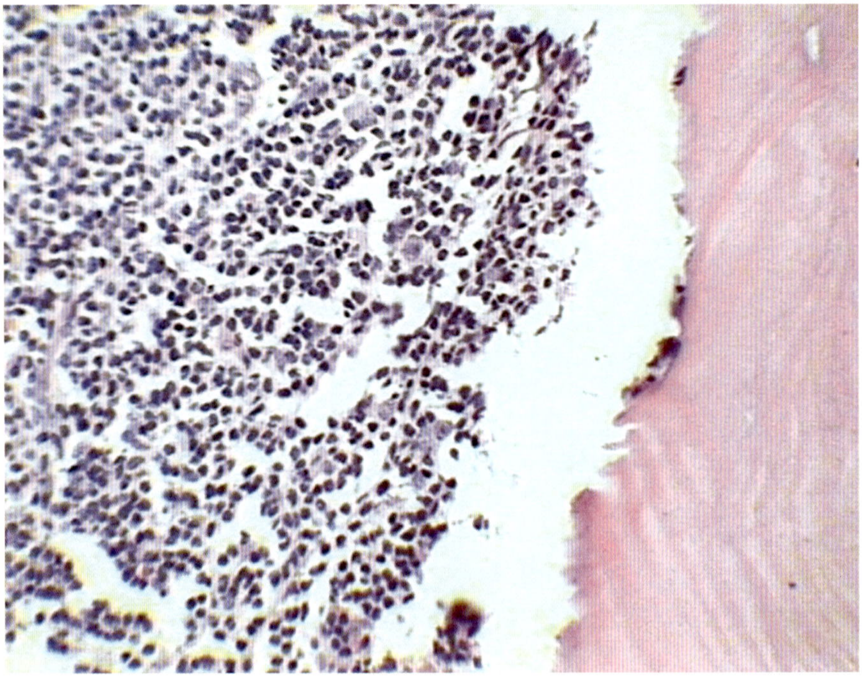

Fig. 6.11: Lymphoma infiltrate—paratrabecular aggregate

Bone marrow biopsy: The bone marrow is often diffusely replaced by small lymphocytes. Other patterns include interstitial or nodular infiltration usually seen earlier in the disease (6.11). The diffuse infiltration suggests a worse prognosis.

Differential Diagnosis

- Lymphomatous involvement of bone marrow—Definitive diagnosis is made by lymph node biopsy
- Reactive lymphocytosis—Diagnosis is clinched by clinical history, morphology of lymphocytes and rarely immunophenotyping is needed to make a final diagnosis (Fig. 6.12).

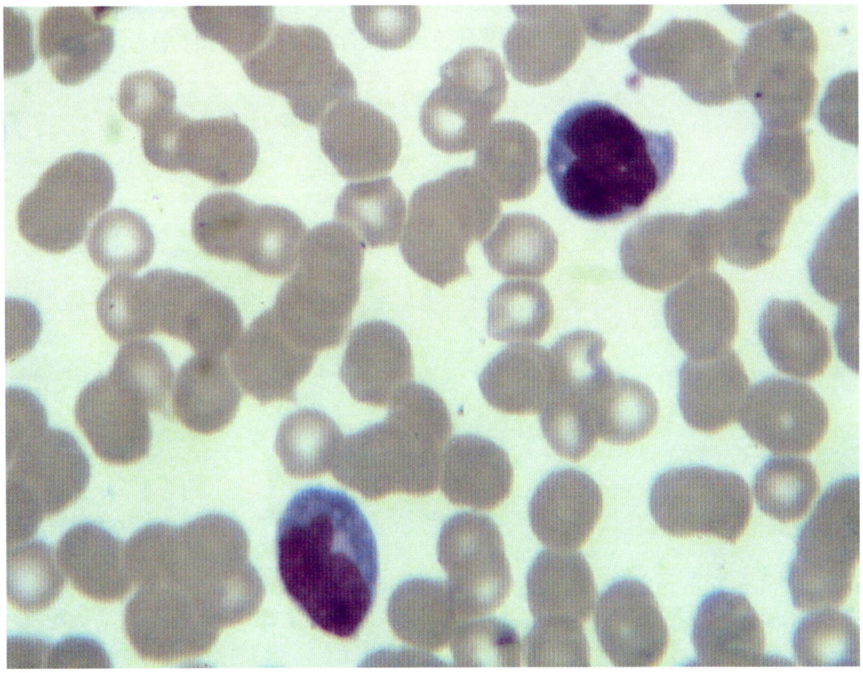

Fig. 6.12: Peripheral smear of a patient with viral infection showing activated lymphocytes—abundant deep basophilic cytoplasm

Clinical Features and Presentation

- Often asymptomatic; lymphocytosis (>5.0 × 10^9/l) on routine FBC
- With more advanced disease: lymphadenopathy: painless, often symmetrical, splenomegaly (66%), hepatomegaly and ultimately BM failure due to infiltration causing anemia, neutropenia and thrombocytopenia
- Recurrent infection due to acquired hypogammaglobulinemia: Especially Herpes zoster
- Patients with advanced disease: weight loss, night sweats, general malaise
- Autoimmune phenomena occur; DAT +ve in 10 to 20 percent cases, warm antibody AIHA in <50 percent cases. Autoimmune thrombocytopenia in 1 to 2 percent.

Treatment

- Patients with asymptomatic lymphocytosis simply require monitoring
- Chemotherapy reserved for patients with symptomatic or progressive disease: anemia (Hb <10g/dL) or thrombocytopenia (<100 x 10^9/l), constitutional symptoms due to CLL (>10% weight loss in 6 months, fatigue, fever, night sweats), progressive lymphocytosis >300 x 10^9/l; doubling time <12 months, symptomatic lymphadenopathy/hepatosplenomegaly, autoimmune disease refractory to steroids, repeated infections
- Many drugs are effective in CLL alone or in combination like chlorambucil, fludarabine, cyclophosphamide, bendamustine, rituximab, etc. Treatment option depends upon age and performance status of the patient and individualized.

CLL remains an incurable disease with current therapy apart from a few allografted patients but most patients with early stage, asymptomatic CLL die of other, unrelated causes.

Prognosis

CLL is an innocuous disease and has a long survival. Its prognostic factors are given in Table 6.2.

Table 6.2: Prognostic factors in CLL

	Low-risk	*High-risk*
Gender	*Female*	*Male*
Clinical stage	Binet A	Binet B and C
	Rai 0,1	2,3,4
Lymphocyte doubling time (LDT)	>12 months	<12 months
Lymphocyte morphology	Typical	Atypical
Pattern of marrow infiltration	Non diffuse	Diffuse
Serum markers	Normal	Increased
B2 microglobulin LDH		>3.5 mg/l
Serum thymedine kinase		>70 u/l
Genetic abnormalities	Normal	11 q-
		17q-
		loss of P53
IgVH gene status	Mutated	Unmutated

CD38 and ZAP 70 are considered as surrogate marker for mutation status.

PROLYMPHOCYTIC LEUKEMIA (PLL) (FIG. 6.13)

This is a rare chronic lymphoproliferative disorder seen in elderly in which patients have high total leukocyte count along with massive splenomegaly. The prolymphocytes are morphologically characterized by a large nucleus with opened up chromatin and a single centrally placed prominent nucleoli (Fig. 6.13). The number of prolymphocytes required for a diagnosis of PLL is 55 percent.

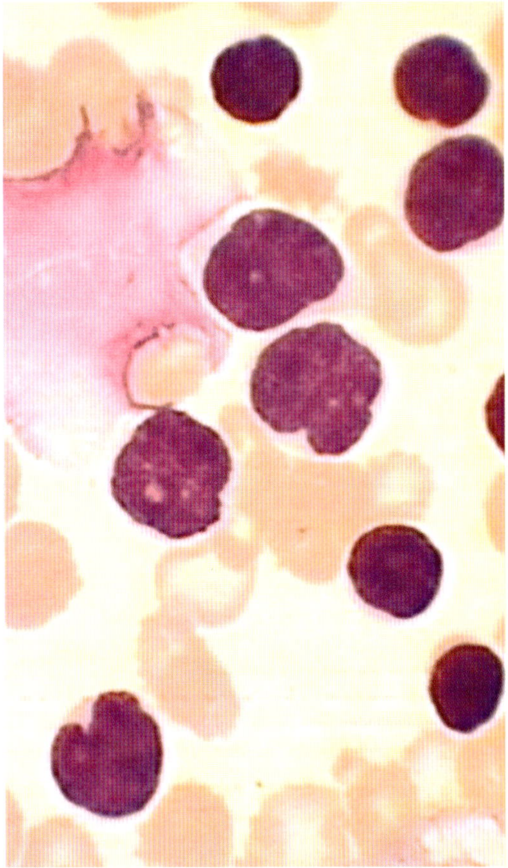

Fig. 6.13: PLL—Peripheral smear showing leukocytosis with prolymphocytes showing large opened out nucleus having prominent nucleolus and scant cytoplasm

HAIRY CELL LEUKEMIA (HCL) (FIGS 6.14 TO 6.17)

This is a chronic lymphoproliferative disorder which unlike PLL present with pancytopenia along with massive splenomegaly. Peripheral smear may show atypical lymphoid cells with hairy projections and blue cytoplasm (Fig. 6.14A). These hairy cells are positive for acid phosphatase which is resistant to tartrate (Fig. 6.14B). A buffy coat preparation for demonstration of hairy cells may be handy in markedly pancytopenic patients.

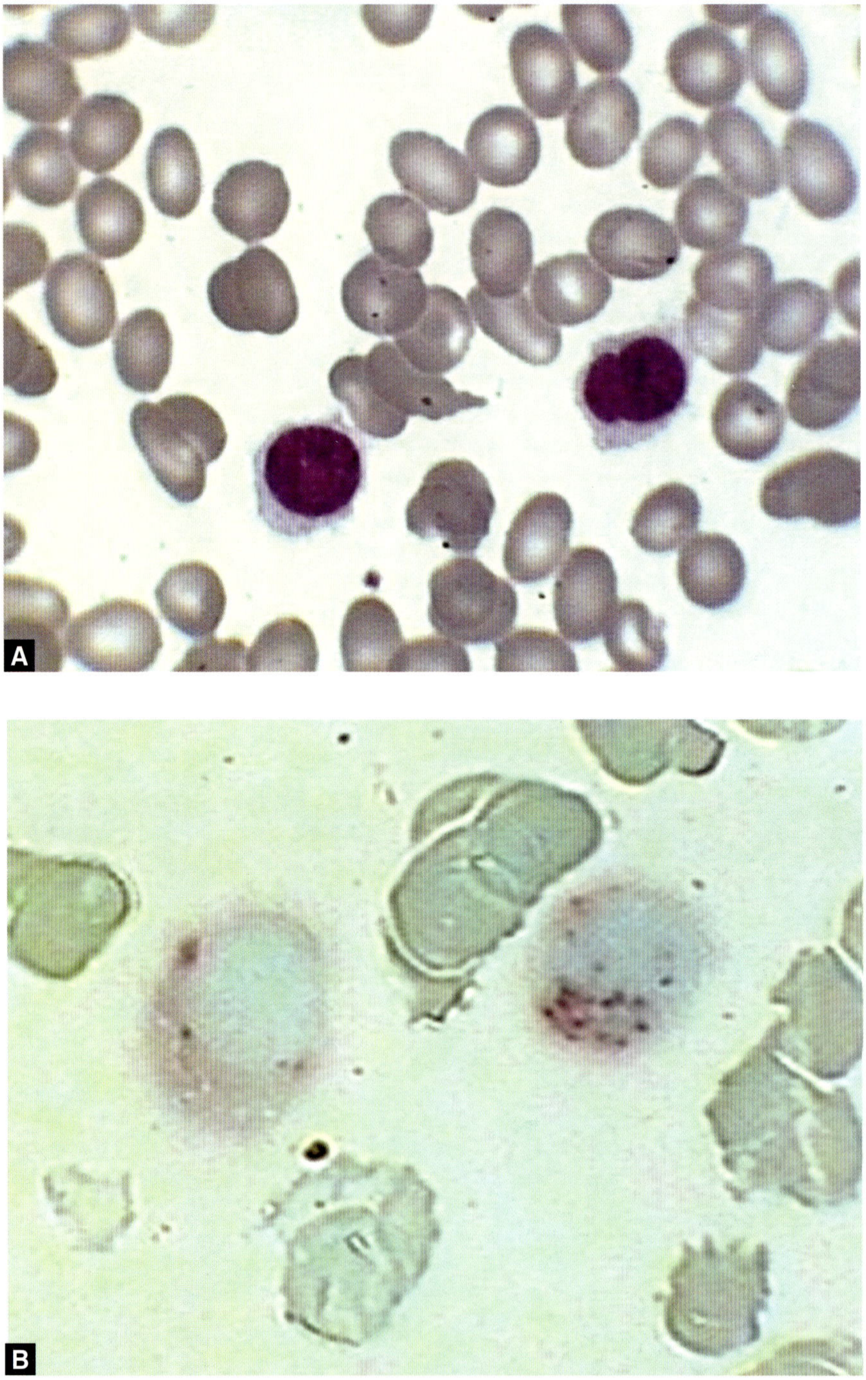

Figs 6.14A and B: (A) Hairy projections on lymphocytes in hairy cell leukemia; (B) Tartarate resistant acid phosphatase positivity (Red granules)

Bone marrow biopsy shows characteristic morphological appearance in the form of "fried egg" or "honey- comb" pattern with clusters of cells with a clear space around them (Fig. 6.15).

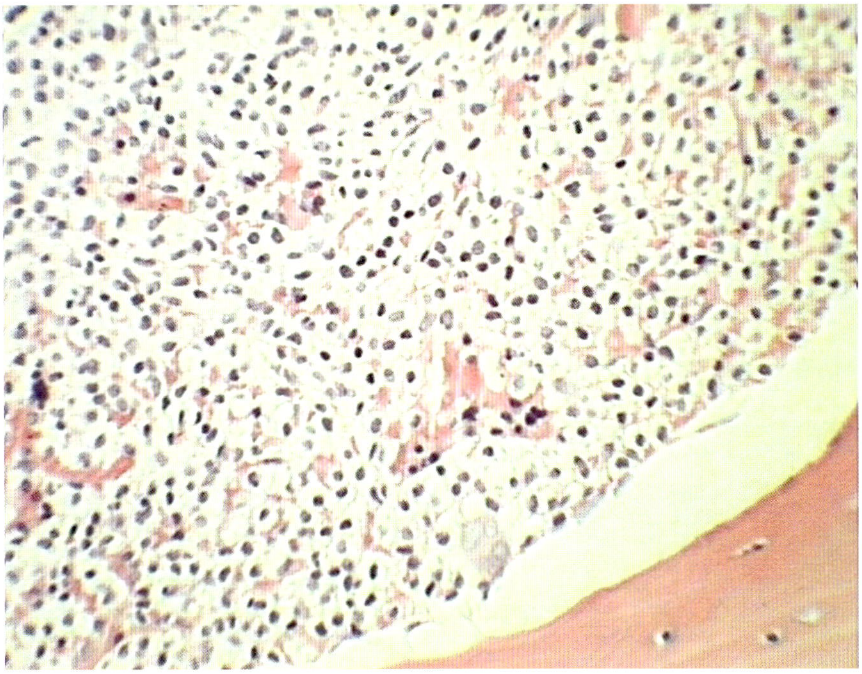

Fig. 6.15: Bone biopsy showing *fried egg* appearance

Electron microscopic morphology is pathognomonic and shows interdigitating hairy like projections both between the microvilli of single cell or between multiple cells (Fig. 6.16A and B).

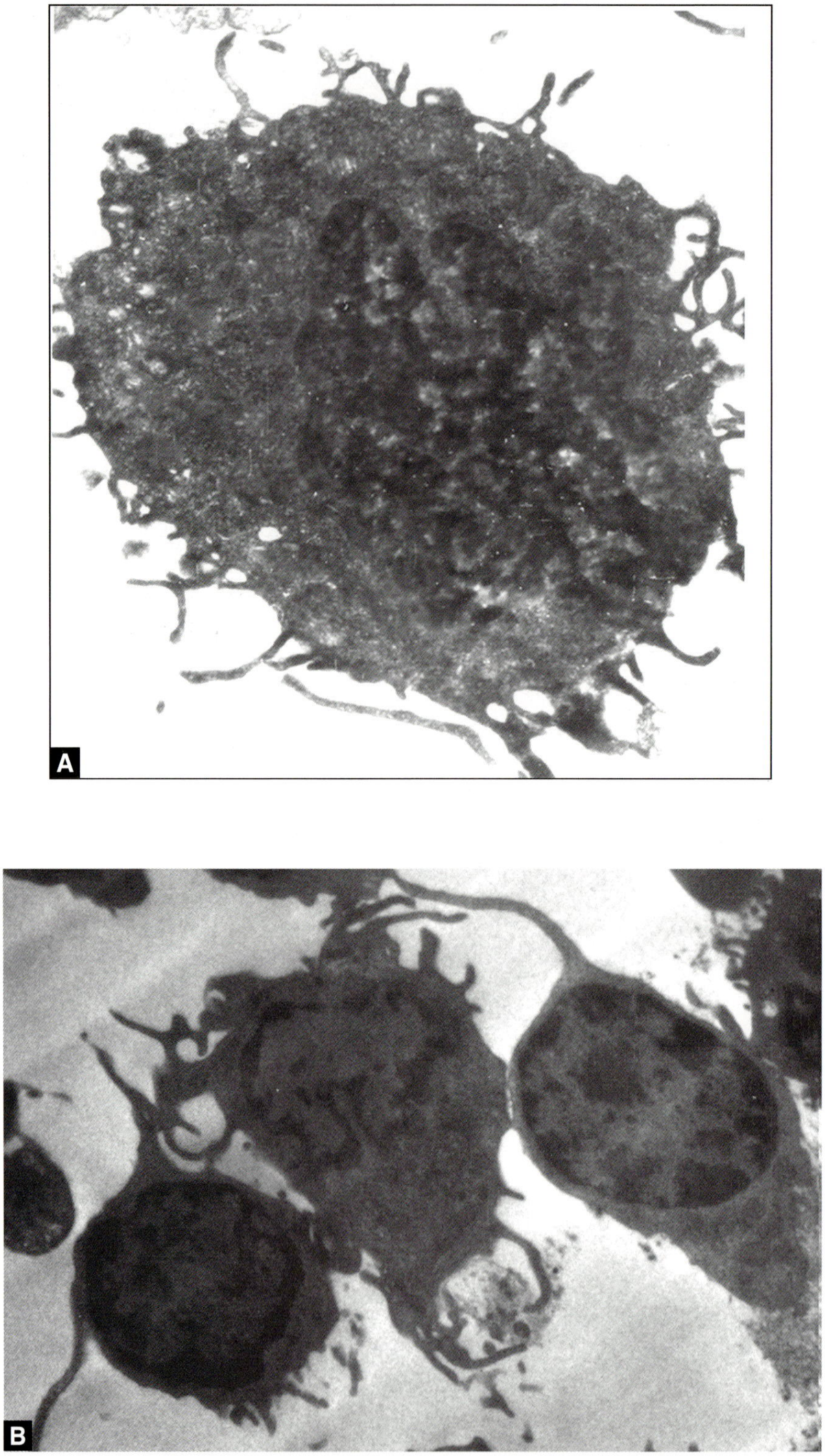

Figs 6.16A and B: (A) Electron microscopy (EM) showing interdigiting villi on surface of lymphocytes; (B) Electron microscopy (EM) showing interdigiting villi between lymphocytes

Ribosomal lamellar complexes are another important diagnostic morphological feature (Fig. 6.17). As with other lymphoproliferative disorders, these may be associated with autoimmune hemolytic anemia.

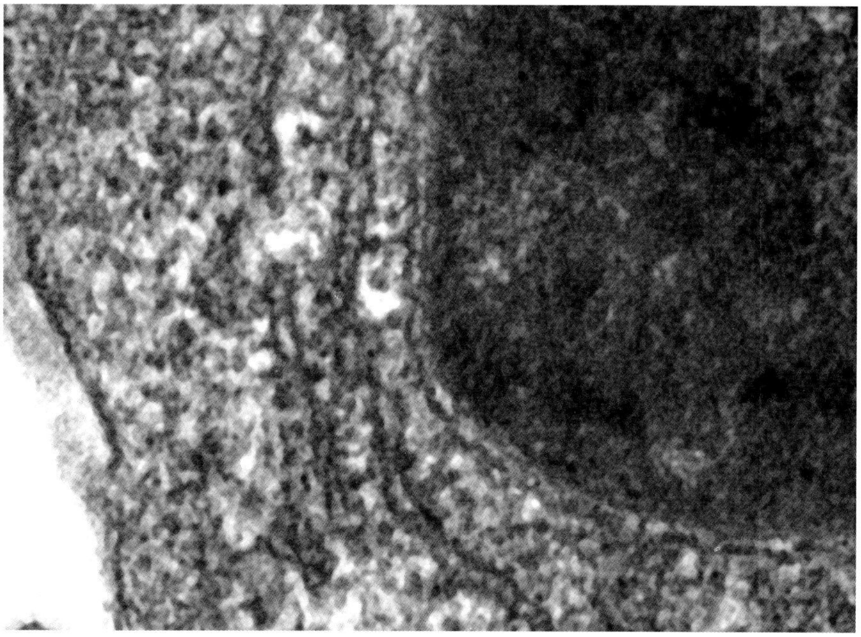

Fig. 6.17: Electron microscopy (EM) showing ribosomal lamellar complexes in lymphocytes

Clinical features: The median age of presentation is between 50 to 55 years. Classically, these patients present with weakness and fatigue. Most patients of HCL have splenomegaly in the absence of peripheral lymphadenopathy and a variable degree of pancytopenia with severe monocytopenia.

Treatment: Patients with HCL may not require treatment for many years, but should be considered for treatment if they are symptomatic or if there is significant pancytopenia. The standard therapy for HCL is with one of the nucleoside analog like dCF or CdA (Cladribine). The usual dose of cladribine: 0.1 mg.kg/day for 7 days.

CHAPTER 7

Myelofibrosis

CHAPTER OVERVIEW

- Introduction
- Myelofibrosis

This is the condition where there is increased reticulin laying down in the bone marrow. This may be seen in tuberculosis, lymphomas, myelodysplastic syndrome, etc. or may be idiopathic. Before labeling it as idiopathic, it is important to exclude acquired causes. The hemogram shows anemia which may be associated with pancytopenia or thrombocytopenia. Rarely there may be associated thrombocytosis. The peripheral smear examination can give a clue to underlying myelofibrosis. It shows leukoerythroblastosis (Fig. 7.1) and presence of fully

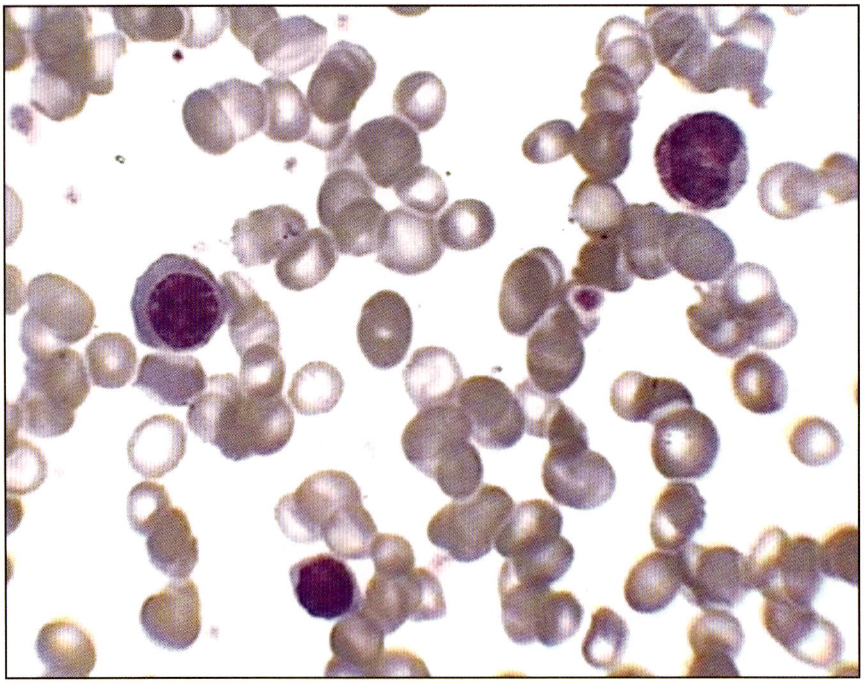

Fig. 7.1: Peripheral smear shows leukoerythroblastic blood picture

hemoglobinated tear drop red cells (Fig. 7.2). Bone marrow aspiration is almost always a dry tap. Bone marrow biopsy, on H and E stains shows megakaryocytic hyperplasia with fibroblastic hyperplasia (Fig. 7.3).

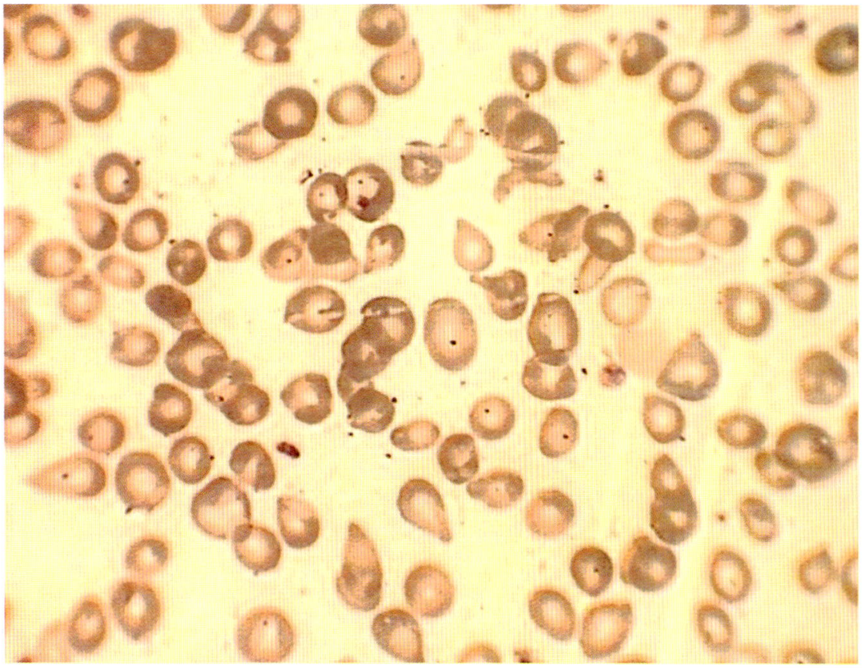

Fig. 7.2: Peripheral smear shows normocytic normochromic red cells with tear drop red cells

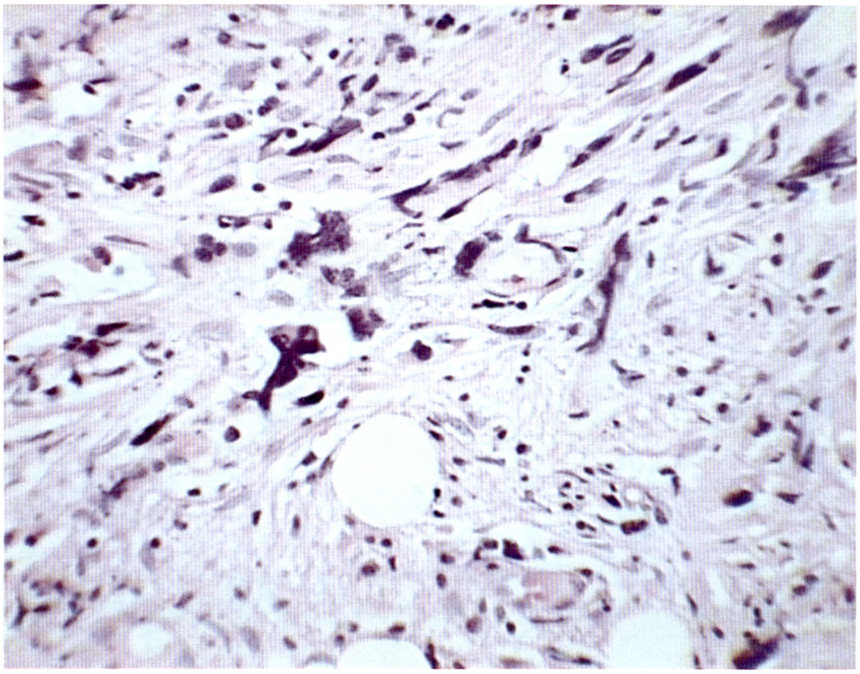

Fig. 7.3: Bone biopsy (H & E stain) showing fibrosis of marrow and increased megakaryocytes

The reticulin stain shows increased reticulin fibers showing grade 2 to 3 positivity (Fig. 7.4). Masson's trichrome stain shows positivity in grade 3 myelofibrosis. It needs to be differentiated from osteopetrosis where there is new bone laying down in the marrow (Fig. 7.5).

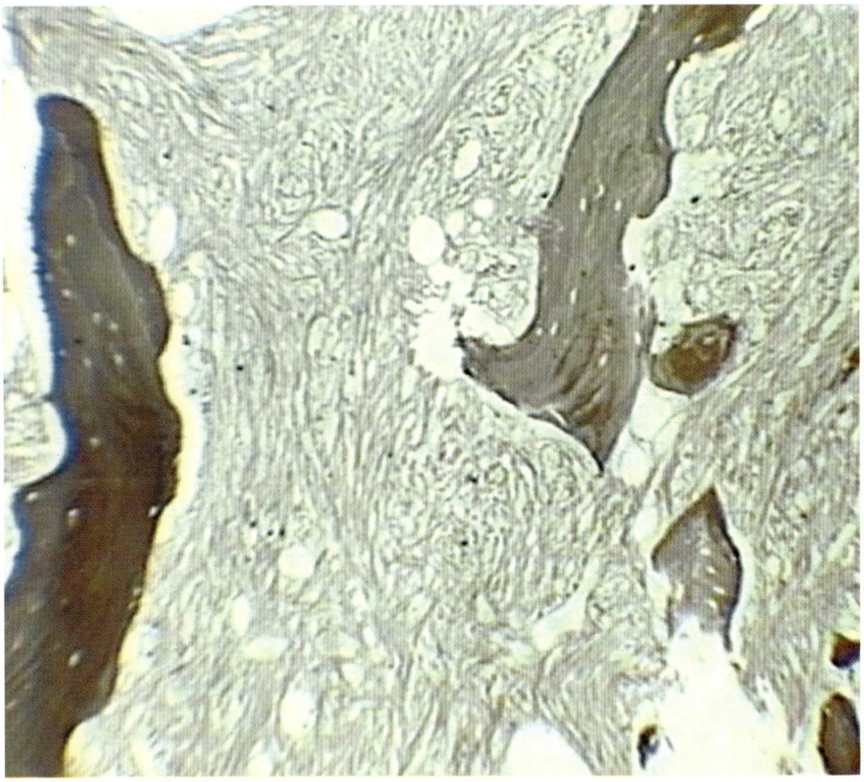

Fig. 7.4: Bone biopsy showing increased reticulin (2 to 3+) (Reticulin stain)

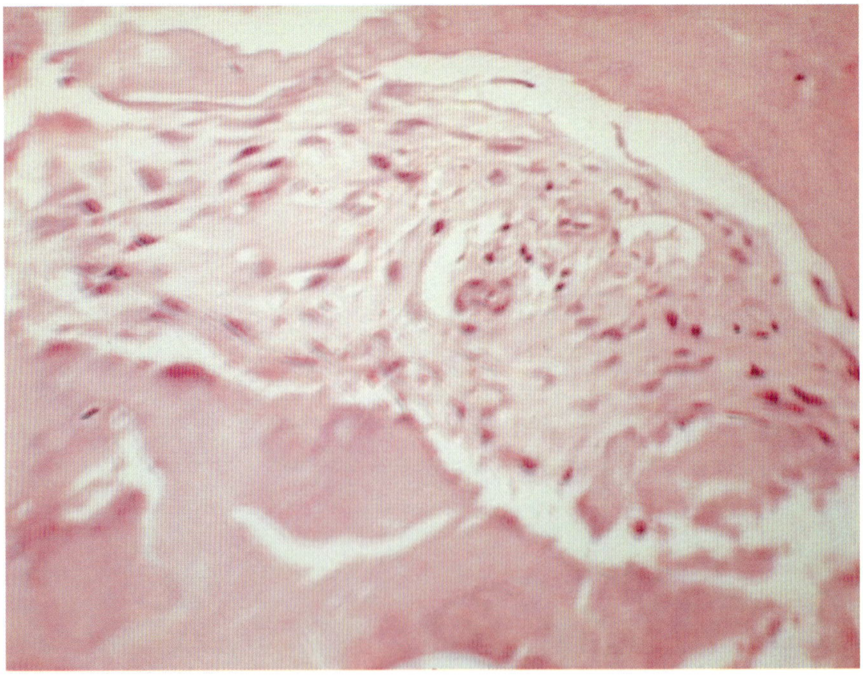

Fig. 7.5: Bone biopsy from a case of osteopetrosis showing increased bone formation in the marrow spaces

Clinical Features and Presentation

- Greater than or equal to 20 percent may be asymptomatic at diagnosis: mild abnormalities identified on routine FBC or splenomegaly at clinical examination
- Most present with symptoms of progressive anemia and hepatosplenomegaly associated with hypercatabolic features of fatigue, weight loss, night sweats and low grade fever
- Abdominal discomfort (heavy sensation in left upper quadrant) and/or dyspepsia from pressure effects of splenic enlargement may prompt presentation
- Symptoms and signs of marrow failure: lethargy, infections, bleeding
- Splenomegaly is almost universal (>90%): moderate to massive (35%) enlargement; variable hepatomegaly (up to 70%); lymphadenopathy is uncommon (<10%)
- Gout in ~5 percent; portal hypertension, pleural effusion and ascites (due to portal hypertension or peritoneal seeding) also occur
- Twenty to thirty percent of patients with PMF are diagnosed in pre-fibrotic stage which clinically mimic ET; proliferation of megakaryocyte with moderate to marked thrombocytosis, mild anemia, mild-to-moderate leukocytosis or modest splenomegaly.

Management

- Myelofibrosis is incurable except by allogeneic SCT but only few patients are eligible; no other treatment alters disease course or prevents leukemic transformation
- Treatment palliative; aiming to improve anemia, alleviate symptomatic organomegaly and hypercatabolic symptoms
- Treatment of anemia—in addition to red cell transfusion, danazol, prednisolone, erythropoietin, etc. has been used with 40 to 50 percent response
- Anti-angiogenic agents like thalidomide or lenalidomide in combination with low dose prednisolone may improve cytopenias and spleen size
- *Cytoreductive therapy:* Hydroxyurea, melphalan, busulfan, etc. to control leukocytosis or thrombocytosis
- Splenectomy indicated for massive or symptomatic splenomegaly, excessive blood transfusion requirements, refractory thrombocytopenia and hypercatabolic symptoms unresponsive to hydroxyurea; evaluate coagulation system preoperatively; 10 percent mortality; 40 percent morbidity
- Splenic irradiation to reduce splenic size and discomfort in those unfit for splenectomy (3–6 months benefit)
- Radiotherapy also a useful treatment of extramedullary hemopoietic infiltrates at other sites, e.g. plueral and peritoneal cavities
- *Allogeneic SCT:* Only therapy for PMF with curative potential. Should be considered for all high risk patients.myeloablative conditioning regimens have been associated with high transplant related mortality(25–48%. Reduced intensity conditioning regimens are less toxic and are being more explored.

Prognosis

- Worst prognosis among Ph-MPNs; median survival 3.5 to 5 years (range 1–30 years)
- Hypersplenism often develops as the spleen enlarges
- Progressive cachexia occurs due to hypercatabolic state in advance IMF. Death in symptomatic cases usually due to infection and hemorrhage
- Around 5 to 10 percent transform to AML refractory to intensive chemotherapy.

CHAPTER 8

Plasma Cell Dyscrasias

CHAPTER OVERVIEW

- ❐ Monoclonal gammopathy of undetermined significance (MGUS)
- ❐ Smoldering myeloma
- ❐ Multiple myeloma
- ❐ Solitary plasmacytoma of the bone
- ❐ Amyloidosis

Plasma cell dyscrasias may be seen in a variety of conditions. These include monoclonal gammopathy of undetermind significance (MGUS), smoldering myeloma and multiple myeloma. However, since increased plasma cells can also be seen in a variety of conditions such as tuberculosis, leishmaniasis and benign monoclonal gammopathy in addition to multiple myeloma, other parameters need to be also consulted before diagnosis, as given below:

Criterion for diagnosis of plasma cell dyscrasia according to Kyle and Grippe.

MONOCLONAL GAMMOPATHY OF UNDETERMINED SIGNIFICANCE (MGUS)

- Serum monoclonal protein (<3 g/dl)
- No anemia, renal failure or hypercalcemia
- Bone lesion absent on radiographic bone surgery
- Bone marrow <10% plasma cells.

SMOLDERING MYELOMA

- Serum monoclonal protein (≥3 g/dl) on >10% marrow plasma cells or aggregates on biopsy or both
- No anemia, renal failure or hypercalcemia attributable myeloma.

MULTIPLE MYELOMA

- Presence of monoclonal plasma cells in bone marrow
- Plus one or more of the following (CRAB*)
  - Anemia
  - Lytic lesions or osteoporosis
  - Renal insufficiency
  - Hypercalcemia

Morphology of plasma cells in multiple myeloma: Typically a large

* C = Calcium (elevated); R = Renal failure; A = Anemia and B = Bone lesions.

number of immature plasma cells are seen along with mature plasma cells (Fig. 8.1). Immature plasma cells have light blue cytoplasm with the frayed out edges and large eccentric nucleus, sometimes with nucleolus. Peri nuclear halo is always there, which help in distinguishing plasma cells from erythroid cells or osteoblasts with which they may sometimes be confused. Presence of syncitial forms of three or more plasma cells clinches the diagnosis of multiple myeloma. Often this is associated with Rouleaux formation in peripheral smear and bluish background in the bone marrow aspirate due to hypergammaglobulinemia (Fig. 8.2).

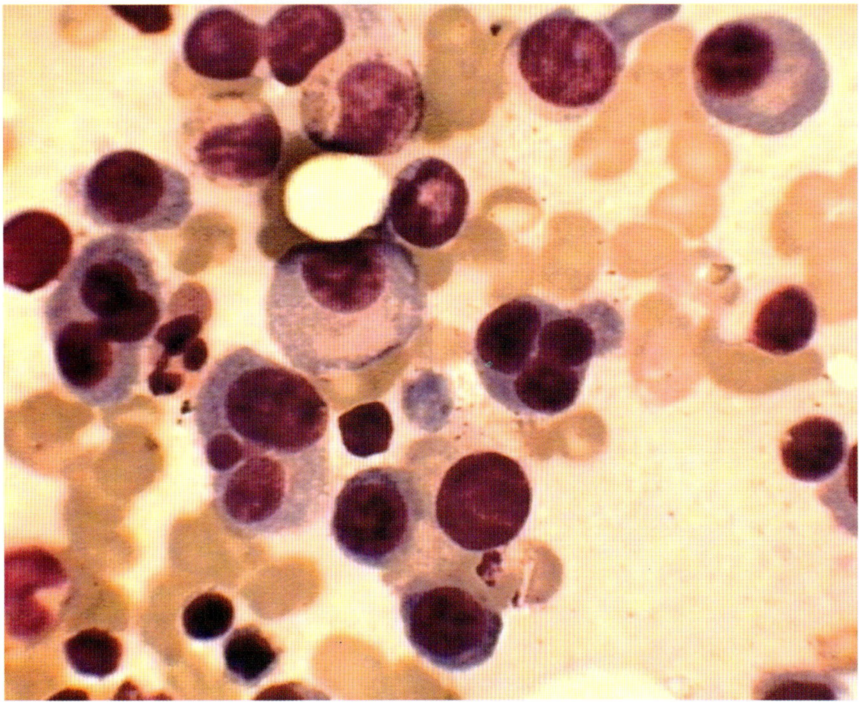

Fig. 8.1: Bone marrow showing immature plasma cells

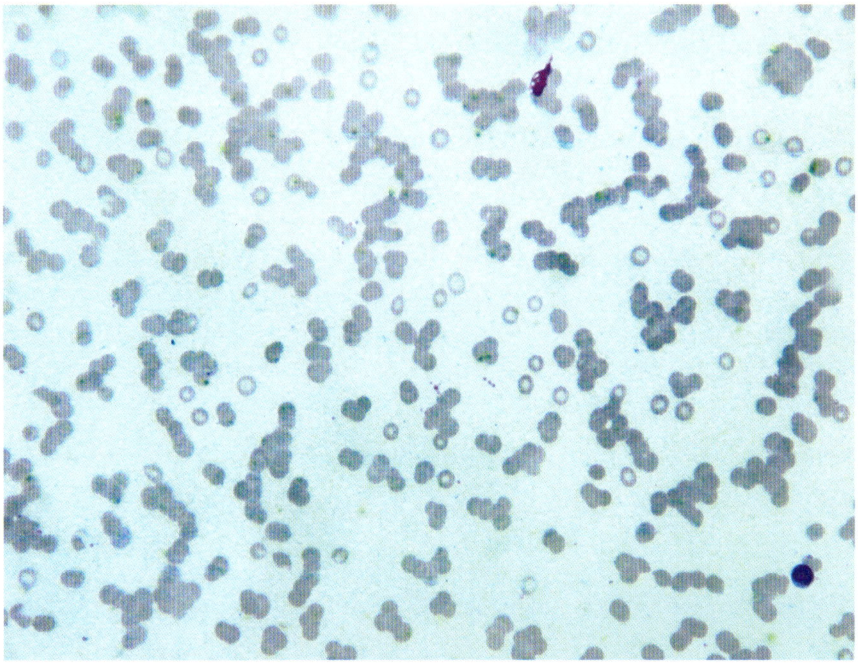

Fig. 8.2: Peripheral smear showing Rouleaux formation

Other disorders with plasma cells which need to be differentiated from multiple myeloma are the following:

Monoclonal gammopathy of uncertain significance (MGUS): This is characterized by presence of

- Serum M protein of <3 g/dl (Fig. 8.3)
- Less than 10% plasma cells in BM
- No or only small amount of Bence Jones protein in urine
- Absence of lytic lesions
- Absence of anemia
- Absence of hypercalcemia
- No renal insufficiency
- Most importantly stability of M protein.

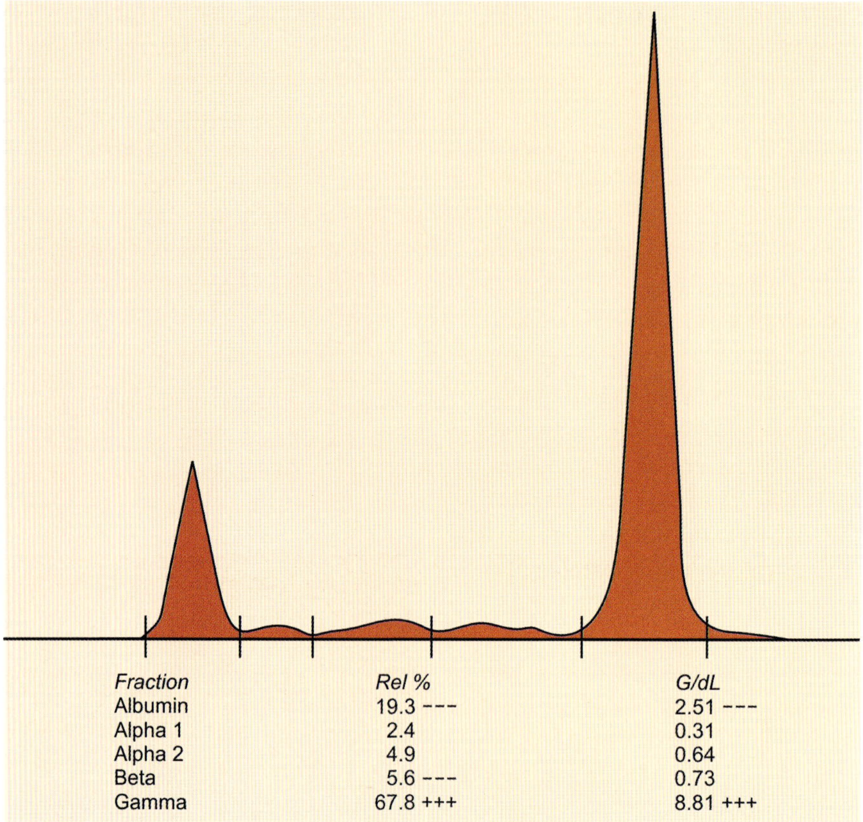

Fig. 8.3: Serum electrophoresis showing 'M' band at gamma region

Note

- Eleven percent progress to MM
- No single test can distinguish MGUS from MM.

Features of MGUS

- β2-Microglobulin and C-reactive protein levels are normal
- CD56 may not be expressed on the plasma cells.

SOLITARY PLASMACYTOMA OF THE BONE

This diagnosis is based on:

- Histologic evidence of a tumor consisting of monoclonal plasma cells with no other lesion on skeletal survey or MRI
- Normal bone marrow
- Absences of a M protein in blood and urine or if present therapy for the solitary lesion should result in disappearance of the M protein
- Uninvolved Igs are usually normal and there is no evidence of anemia or hypercalcemia.

AMYLOIDOSIS

The following criteria help to differentiate other disorders with monoclonal proteins from multiple myeloma.

Clinical Features and Presentation

- Spectrum from asymptomatic paraproteinemia detected on routine testing (~20%) to rapidly progressive illness with extensive, destructive bony disease
- Most present with bone (usually back) pain (~75%) or pathological fracture; kyphosis and loss of height may occur from vertebral compression fractures
- Weakness and fatigue (>50%), recurrent infection (10%), thirst, polyuria, nocturia or edema due to renal impairment (~10%) also common
- Acute hypercalcemia, symptomatic hyperviscosity (mental slowing, visual upset, purpura, hemorrhage), neuropathy, spinal cord compression, amyloidosis and coagulopathy less frequent at presentation
- There are two important variants of myeloma, solitary bone plasmacytoma and extramedullary plasmacytoma. These lesions are associated with an M component in fewer than 30 percent of the cases, they may affect younger individuals, and both are associated with median survivals of 10 or more years. Solitary bone plasmacytoma is a single lytic bone lesion without marrow plasmacytosis (Fig. 8.3). Extramedullary plasmacytomas usually involve the submucosal lymphoid tissue of the nasopharynx or paranasal sinuses without marrow plasmacytosis. Both tumors are highly responsive to local radiation therapy. Solitary bone plasmacytomas may recur in other bony sites or evolve into myeloma. Extramedullary plasmacytomas rarely recur or progress (Fig. 8.4).

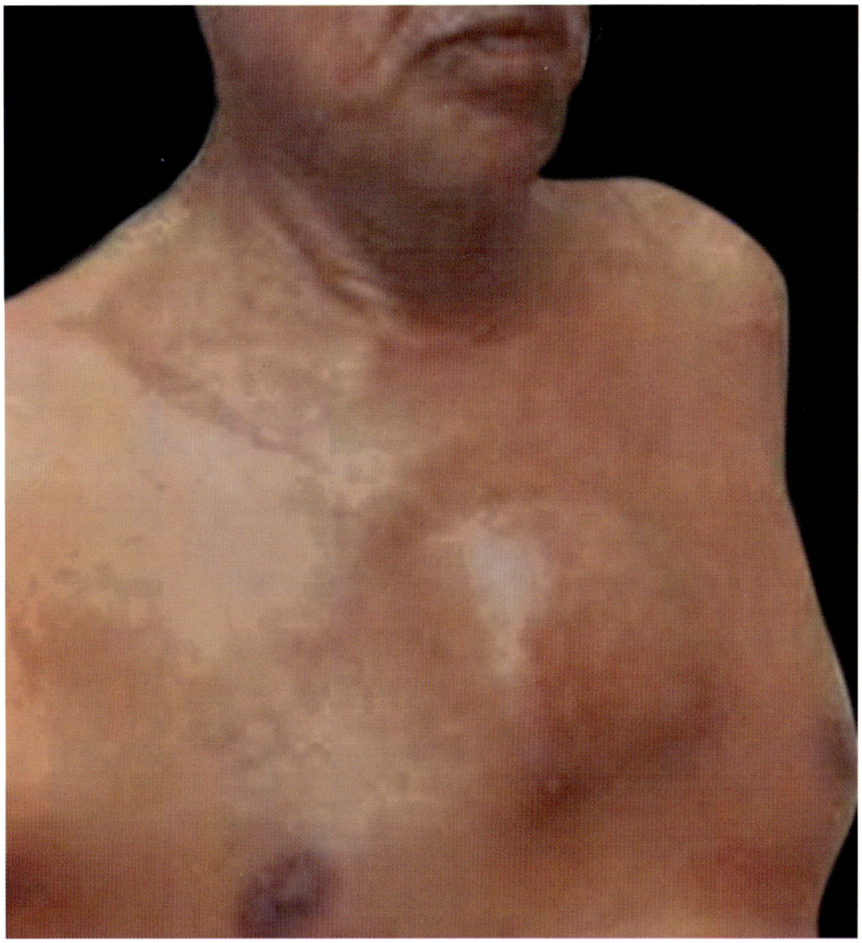

Fig. 8.4: Solitary plasmacytoma of sternum

Investigations in a Case of Suspected Myeloma

- Diagnosis
- BM aspirate demonstrates plasma cell infiltration—may be only way to diagnose non-secretory (NS) myeloma
- Radiological skeletal survey—Identifies lytic lesions (Figs 8.5 and 8.6), fractures and osteoporosis (80%; 5–10% osteoporosis only; 20% normal)
- Paraprotein immunofixation and densitometry—Characterizes and quantifies paraprotein (IgG ~55%; IgA ~22% IgD ~2%; IgM 0.5%; IgE <0.01%; LC ~22%).

Tests to Establish Tumor Burden and Prognosis

- Serum β_2-microglobulin—Measure of tumor load
- Serum C-reactive protein—Surrogate measure of IL-6 which correlates with tumor aggression
- Serum LDH—Measure of tumor aggression
- Serum albumin—Hypoalbuminemia correlates with poor prognosis
- BM cytogenetics.

Treatment

The treatment of myeloma is rapidly changing, with several new active drugs recently developed and approved. The initial step in treatment, referred to as "induction" has changed from being based on cytotoxic chemotherapy to being based on other biologic agents.

Thalidomide, one of the immunomodulatory agents (IMIDs) in combination with dexamethasone

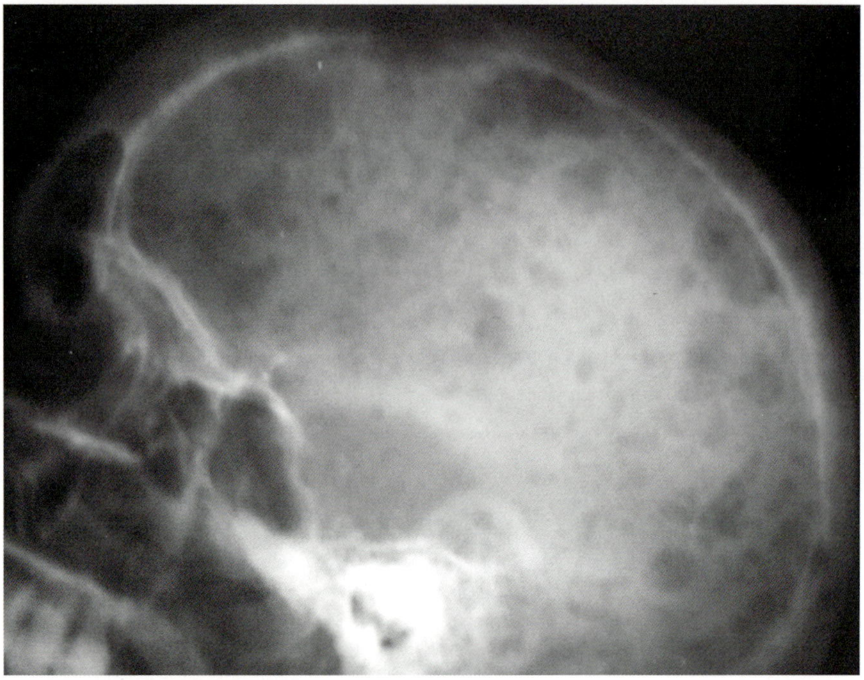

Fig. 8.5: X-ray skull showing multiple lytic lesions suggestive of multiple myeloma

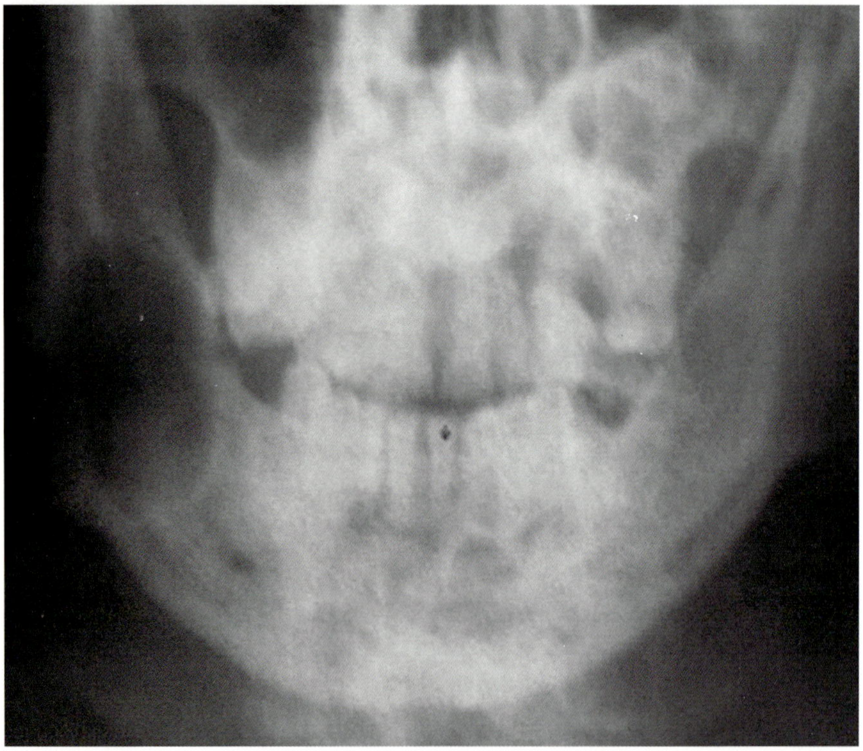

Fig. 8.6: X-ray of jaw bones showing large lytic lesion at the angle of right mandible

was a standard induction treatment until recently. The second-generation agent lenalidomide is both more active and less toxic than thalidomide and is replacing the older drug in treatment. The major side effect of lenalidomide is cumulative myelosuppression.

Bortezomib, a proteosome inhibitor, is also highly active and has the advantages of producing rapid responses and of being effective in poor prognosis myeloma. The major side effect of bortezomib is neuropathy (both peripheral and autonomic), and it has the disadvantage of requiring frequent intravenous administration.

At the present time, induction therapy should include dexamethasone and either lenalidomide or bortezomib or both.

After induction therapy, the optimal consolidation therapy for patients under age 70 years with myeloma is autologous stem cell transplantation. Early aggressive treatment prolongs both duration of remission and overall survival, and has the advantage of providing long treatment-free intervals. Clinical trials are evaluating the role of post transplant maintenance therapy with agents such as lenalidomide.

Allogeneic transplantation is potentially curative in myeloma, but its role has been limited because of the unusually high mortality rate (40–50%) in myeloma patients.

Localized radiotherapy may be useful for palliation of bone pain or for eradicating tumor at the site of pathologic fracture. Hypercalcemia should be treated aggressively and immobilization and dehydration avoided. The bisphosphonates (pamidronate 90 mg or zoledronic acid 4 mg intravenously monthly) reduce pathologic fractures in patients with significant bony disease and are an important adjunct in this subset of patients. However, long-term zoledronate has been associated with a risk of osteonecrosis of the jaw, and patients must be monitored for this complication.

Prognosis

The outlook for patients with myeloma has been steadily improving for the past decade. The median survival of patients is now between four and six years, and it is possible that the use of newly approved agents will result in further survival gains. Novel approaches, possibly involving allogeneic stem cell transplantation, are being studied to try to improve the outlook for patients with high-risk disease.

CHAPTER 9

Infections

CHAPTER OVERVIEW

- Septicemia
- Hemophagocytosis
- Malaria
- Microfilaria
- Tuberculosis

Infections are common in India. These can alter hematological parameters. The following infections may be seen:

SEPTICEMIA

Septicemia is commonly seen in immunocompromised patients. Peripheral smear in such a case shows marked neutrophilic leukocytosis with neutrophils having toxic granules (Fig. 9.1).

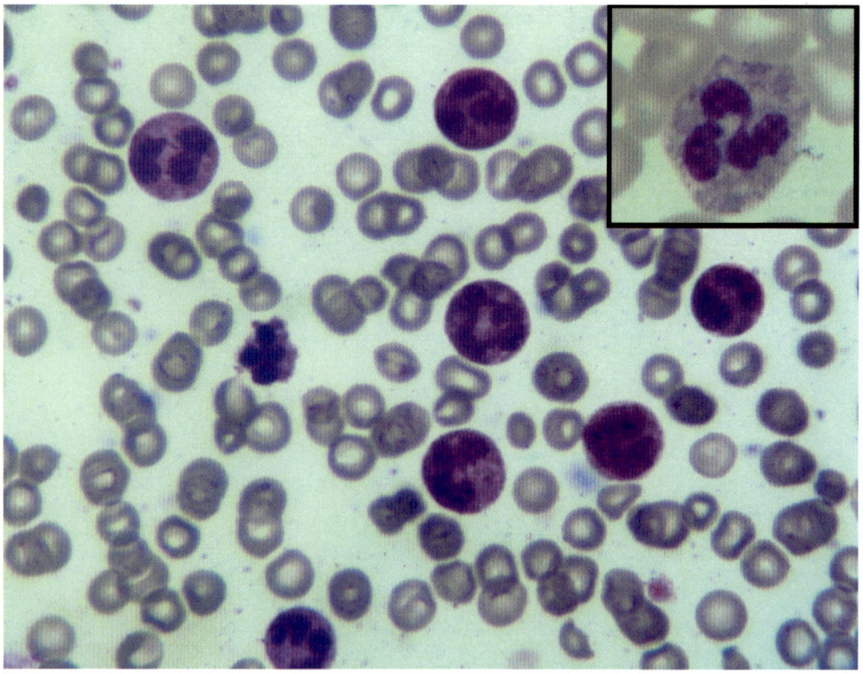

Fig. 9.1: Neutrophilic leukocytosis (Inset: Neutrophil showing toxic granulation)

HEMOPHAGOCYTOSIS

Monocyte-macrophage system cells phagocytosing the hematopoietic cell component is termed as hemophagocytosis. Phagocytic activity restricted to erythroid cells and lymphoid cells is termed as erythrophagocytosis and lymphophagocytosis respectively. The phagocytosing histiocytes usually contain abundant vacuolated cytoplasm, with one or several red blood cells or remnants and containing round to oval nuclei with lacy bland chromatin and inconspicuous nucleoli. Hemophagocytic activity in the bone marrow is seen in a variety of conditions ranging from reactive to neoplastic and can be broadly categorized as below:

a. *Infection associated hemophagocytic syndromes:* It is a non-neoplastic systemic proliferation of benign appearing histiocyte affecting almost every organ including the bone marrow.
b. *Familial hemophagocytic lymphohistiocytosis (FEL)* (Figs 9.2 and 9.3)*:* It is a rare autosomal recessive condition that usually manifests before five years of age with hepatosplenomegaly, fever, pleural effusion, skin rash and usually has a fatal outcome. Pancytopenia, severe hypofibrinogenemia without abnormalities of other clotting factors, increased serum ferritin, increased serum triglycerides are typical laboratory findings. Lymphnodes and the bone marrow are the most frequently involved organs followed by the spleen, liver and CNS. The bone marrow in patients with FEL is partially to

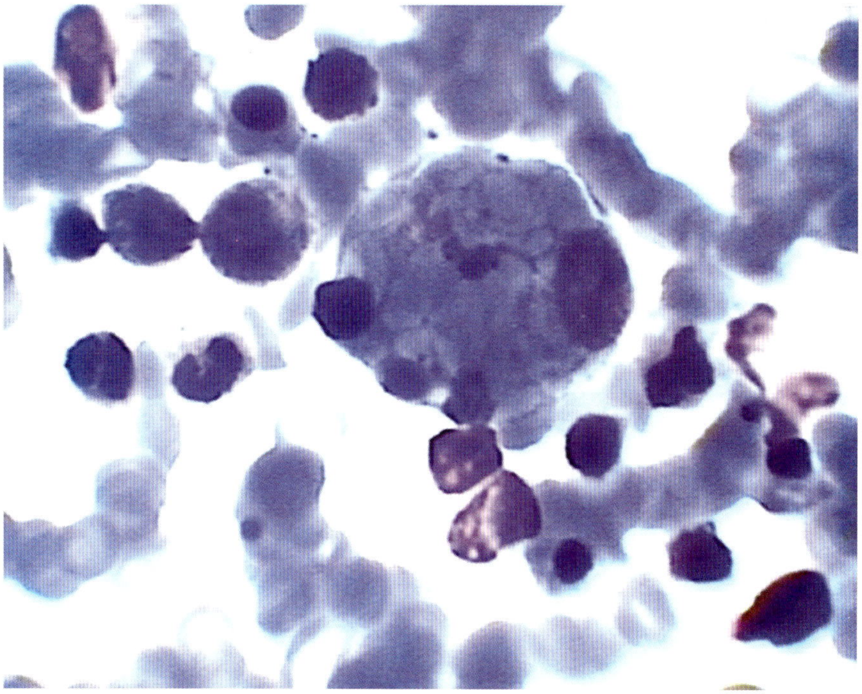

Fig. 9.2: Bone marrow showing hemophagocytosis

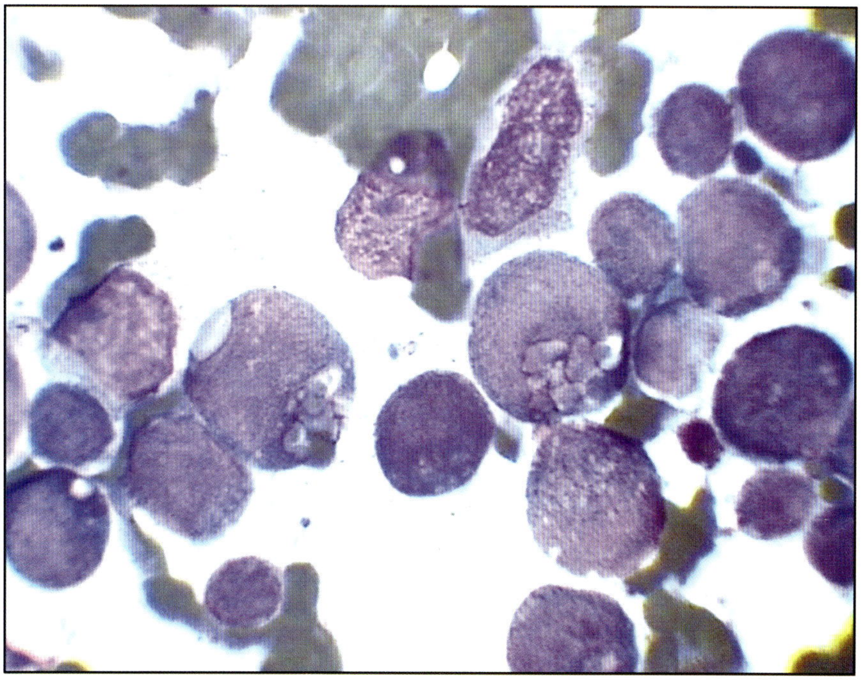

Fig. 9.3: Bone marrow showing blasts with hemophagocytosis

completely effaced by a loose infiltrate of benign appearing histiocytes, lymphocytes and plasma cells. The histiocytosis is quite pronounced and is accompanied by prominent erythrophagocytosis as well as phagocytosis of lymphocytes and other cellular debris. The basic underlying defect in FEL is thought to be a mutation in the Perforin gene. The presently followed diagnostic criteria for hemophagocytic lymphohistiocytosis is given in Table 9.1.

Table 9.1: Diagnostic criteria for hemophagocytic lymphohistiocytosis

Clinical and laboratory criteria (five of eight criteria)
• Family history (seen in familial)
• Fever
• Splenomegaly
• Cytopenia greater than or equal to two cell lines
– Hemoglobin <9.0 g/dl (below 4 weeks <10.0 g/dl)
– Platelets <100 × 10^9/L
– Neutrophils <1.0 × 10^9/L
• Hypertriglyceridemia and/or hypofibrinogenemia (fasting triglycerides >mmol/L; fibrinogen <1.5 g/L)
– Ferritin >500 µg/L
– sCD 25 >2400 U/ml
– Decreased or absent natural killer cell activity
– Hemophagocytosis in bone marrow, CSF or lymph nodes

Storage Disorders

i. *Gaucher's disease:* The enzymatic defect is glucocerebrosidase and the unwanted substrate accumulated in macrophages is glucocerebroside which result in the formation of Gaucher cells. These cells are large round or oval cells with a small, usually eccentric nucleus and voluminous weakly basophilic cytoplasm with a wrinkled or fibrillar or *onion skin* or *crumpled silk* pattern (Figs 9.4 and 9.5).

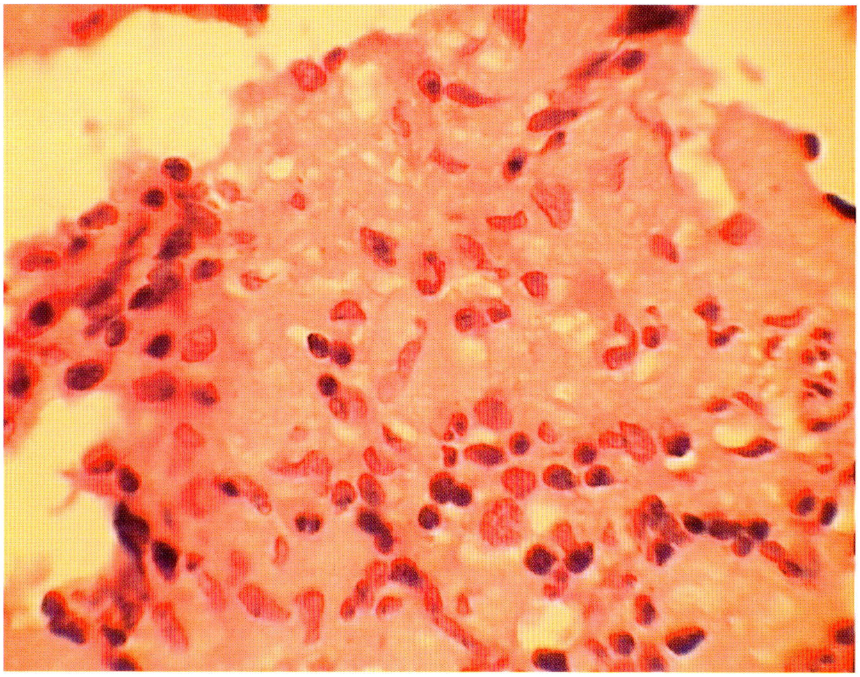

Fig. 9.4: Bone marrow showing a number of cells with large amount of crumpled filter paper type cytoplasm (Gaucher cells)

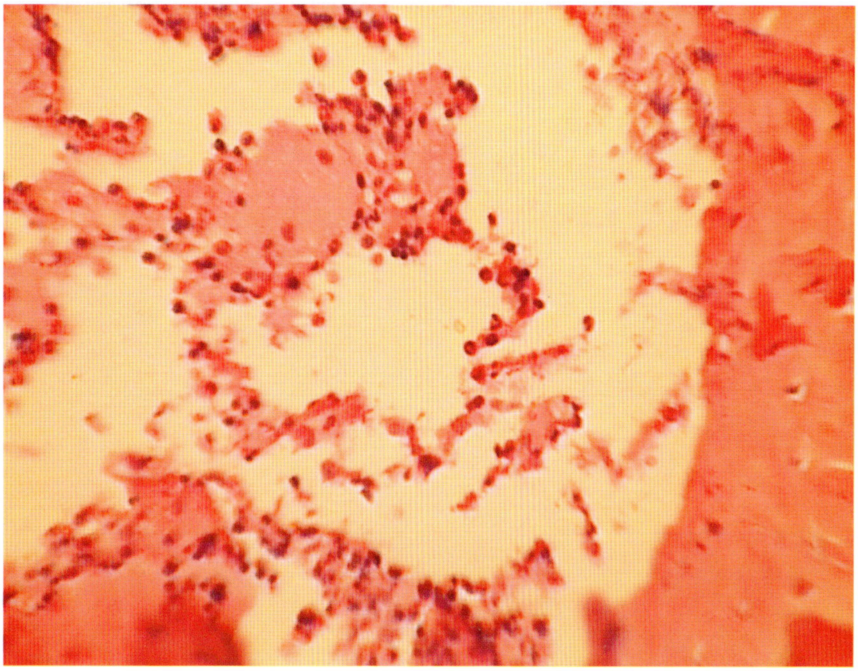

Fig. 9.5: Bone marrow biopsy showing Gaucher cells (Oil immersion microscope)

The cells stain with Sudan black and PAS. They are also TRAP positive and may be positive for iron. Patients with Gaucher's disease may also have an increase in foamy macrophages, the cells which resemble typical Gaucher cells but also contain more strongly basophilic granules. Histological sections of bone marrow biopsy show Gaucher cells in clumps or sheets sometimes replacing large areas of the marrow. The cells have abundant pale staining cytoplasm with a texture that has been likened to watered silk or crumpled tissue paper. There may be an increase in reticulin and collagen deposition. An important morphological differential of a Gaucher cell is a Pseudo-Gaucher cell. These are cells resembling Gaucher cells but not identical to them on ultrastructural examination and are seen in bone marrow in a variety of hematological conditions in which they result from an abnormal load of glucocerebroside presented to macrophages. They are seen in CML, acute leukemia, thalassemia major and CDA and have been recognized in occasional patient with Hodgkin's disease, NHL and a variety of other conditions. Morphologically similar cells have been seen in multiple myeloma and in lymphoplasmacytoid lymphoma but the macrophages in these cases contain material derived from immunoglobulin rather than glucocerebroside. Cells considered to resemble Gaucher cells have also been reported in the bone marrow of a patient with atypical mycobacterial infection complicating AIDS in which the abnormal morphology is due to large numbers of mycobacteria packing the macrophage cytoplasm rather than due to storage of breakdown product.

ii. *Niemann-Pick disease (Fig. 9.6):* The basic enzyme deficient in this disorder is sphingomyelinase and the unwanted substrate accumulated is sphingomyelin. The bone marrow cytology shows foamy macrophages which are large exceeding 50 μ in diameter with

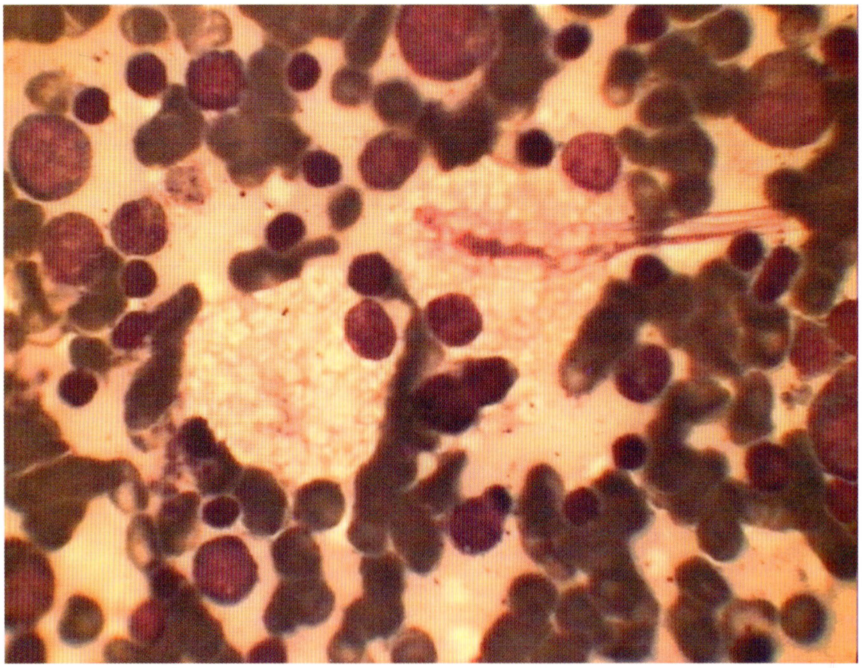

Fig. 9.6: Niemann-Pick cells with vacuolated cytoplasm

a nucleus which is usually central. They stain pale blue with Romanowsky stains and variable with PAS and lipid stains like Oil Red O.

There are also increased numbers of sea blue histiocytes possibly reflecting slow conversion of sphingomyelin to ceroid. Bone marrow histology shows clumps or sheets of foam cells which appear green on Giemsa and light brown on H & E stain; they are PAS positive and usually positive for iron stain.

iii. *Other causes of foamy macrophages in bone marrow:* Other metabolic defects which lead to presence of increased number of foamy macrophages in the bone marrow include hypercholesterolemia, Wolman's disease, Fabry's disease, neuronal lipofuscinosis, Tangier's disease. In Fabry's disease, the storage cells have small globular inclusion which are weakly basophilic on a Romanowsky stain and lightly eosinophilic on H & E. They are PAS negative and SBB-positive. Foam cells are also increased as a result of damage to fat cells including trauma, fat necrosis, bone marrow infarction, infection, previous performance of a bone marrow biopsy of the same site.

- *Sea-blue histiocytosis (Fig. 9.7):* Histiocytic prominence in bone marrow is seen in many reactive conditions like infections, chronic inflammatory disorders and also in benign and malignant histiocytic neoplasms. Apart from the above mentioned disease

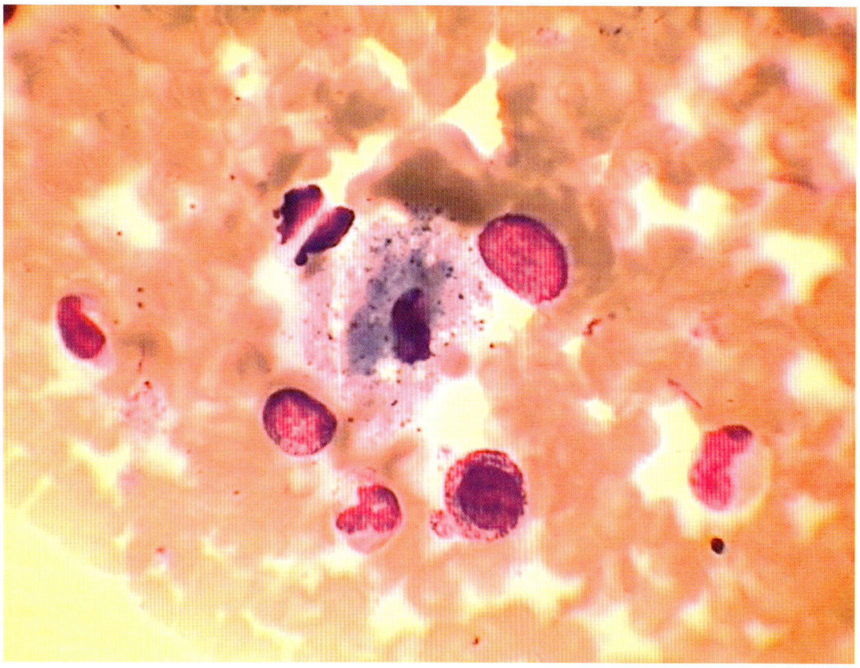

Fig. 9.7: BM aspirate showing sea-blue histiocyte with cytoplasm having inky blue granules

states, a condition called "sea-blue " histiocytosis is existent.This disorder is an inherited condition characterized by presence of sea-blue histiocytes with distinctive morphology containing ceroid or lipofuscin in the bone marrow, liver and spleen. The designation of the disease derives from the staining characteristics of the storage cells on a Ramonowsky stain.

On unstained smears ceroid is brown. Bone marrow cytology shows sea-blue histiocytes stained blue or blue green on a Ramonowsky stain and sometimes positive for iron. Bone marrow histology shows clusters of sea-blue histiocytes as brownish-yellow on H&E stain and blue on a Giemsa stain. They are PAS positive and iron stain positive. They are also acid fast and exhibit autofluorescence.

Other causes of sea-blue histiocytosis: Increased number of sea-blue histiocytes are seen in the bone marrow in a great variety of conditions including many of the conditions in which pseudo-Gaucher's cells are present or foamy macrophages are increased.

- *Leishmaniasis, histoplasmosis:* Bone marrow may show intracellular or extracellular LD bodies. LD bodies can be differentiated from histoplasma since they have a kinetoplast (Figs 9.8 and 9.9).

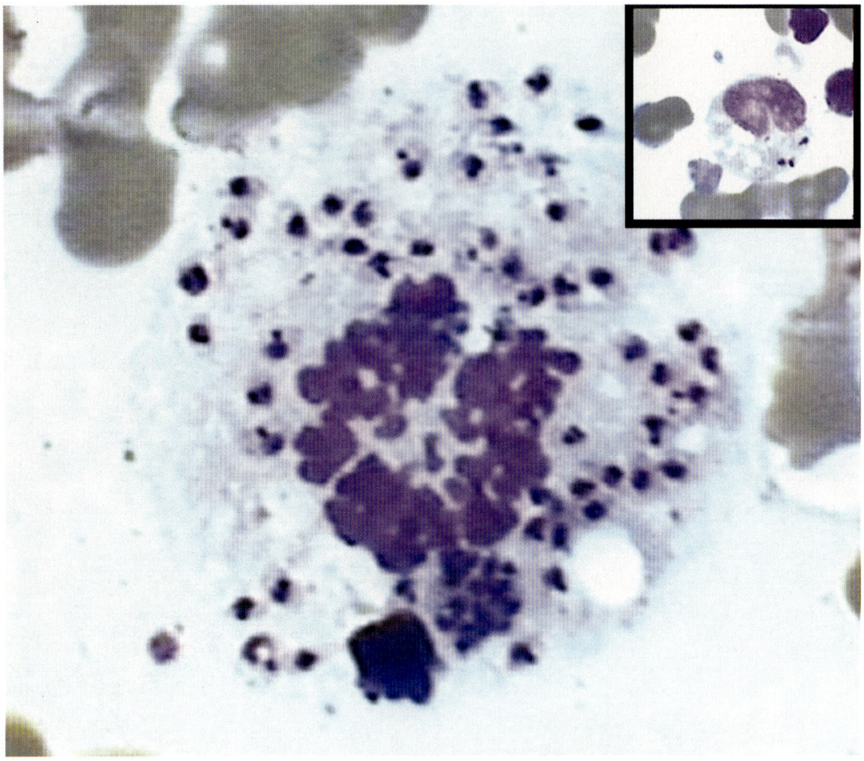

Fig. 9.8: LD bodies showing kinetoplast

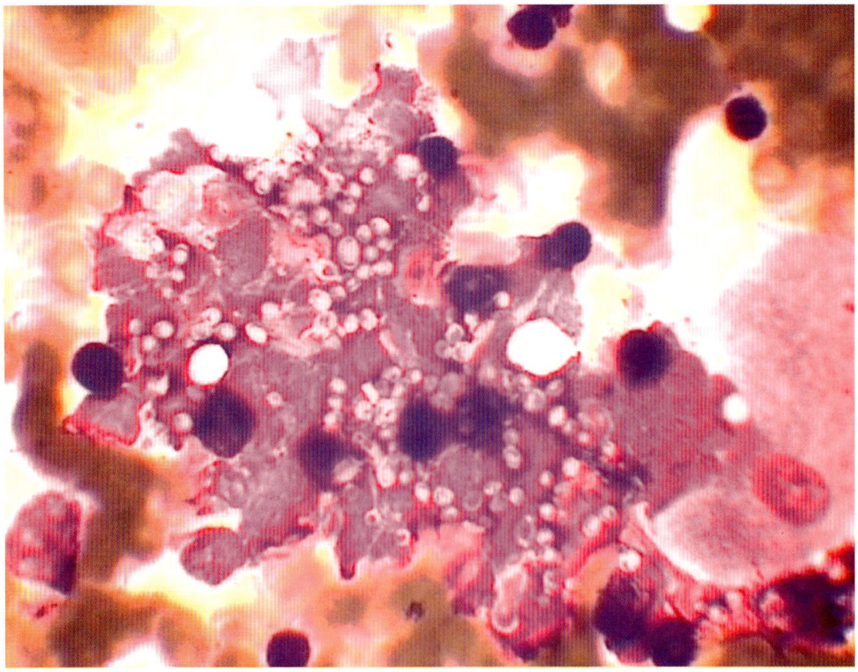

Fig. 9.9: Histoplasma capsulatum

MALARIA

Peripheral blood may show trophozoites/ring forms in *P vivax* or gametocytes in *P falciparum* (Figs 9.10 and 9.11).

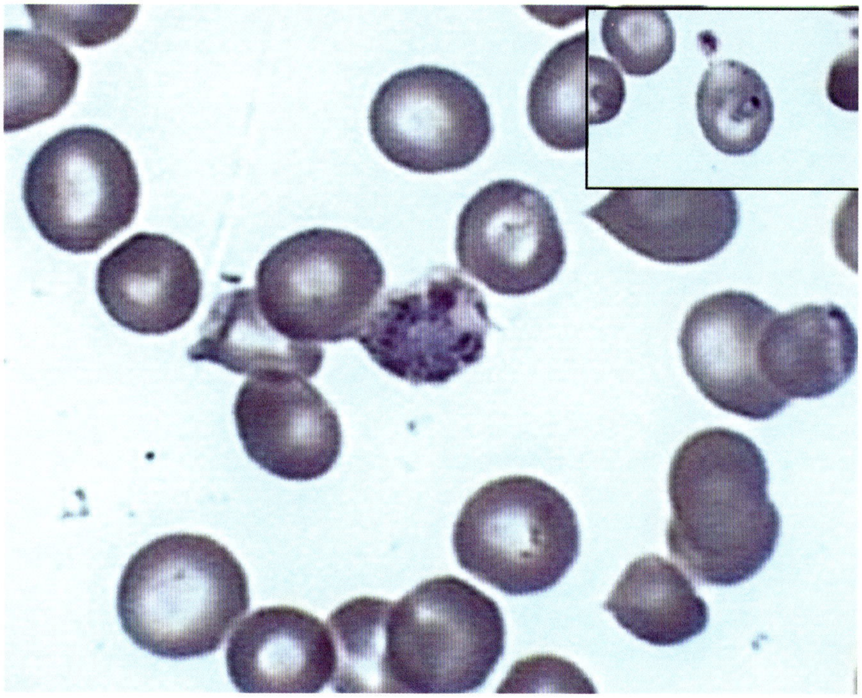

Fig. 9.10: *P vivax* trophozoites

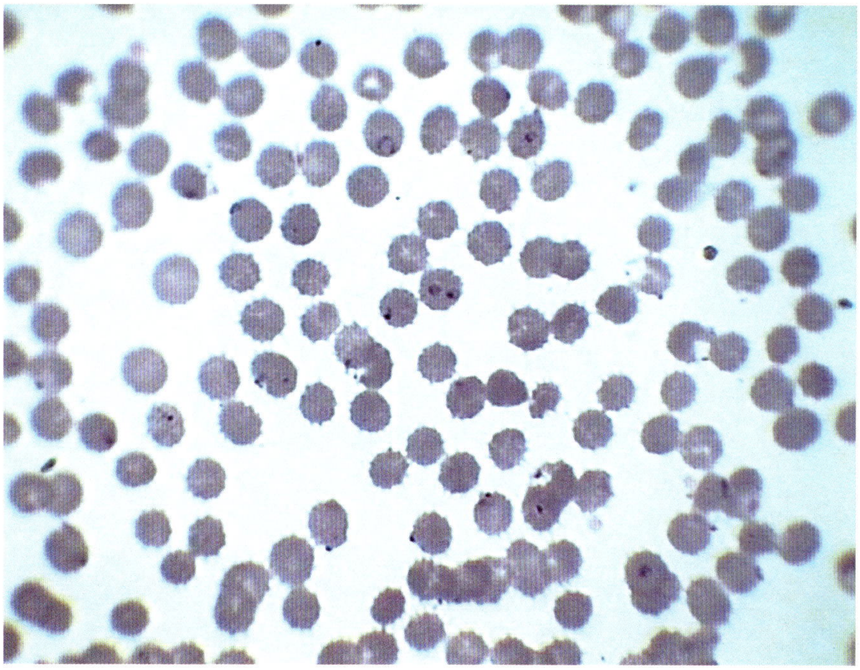

Fig. 9.11: Heavy parasitemia *P. falciparum* rings

MICROFILARIA

Sometimes peripheral smear in patient with fever may show presence of microfilaria. This is specially seen at thick edges. Thus, a peripheral smear should be scanned at 10X to pick it up (Fig. 9.12).

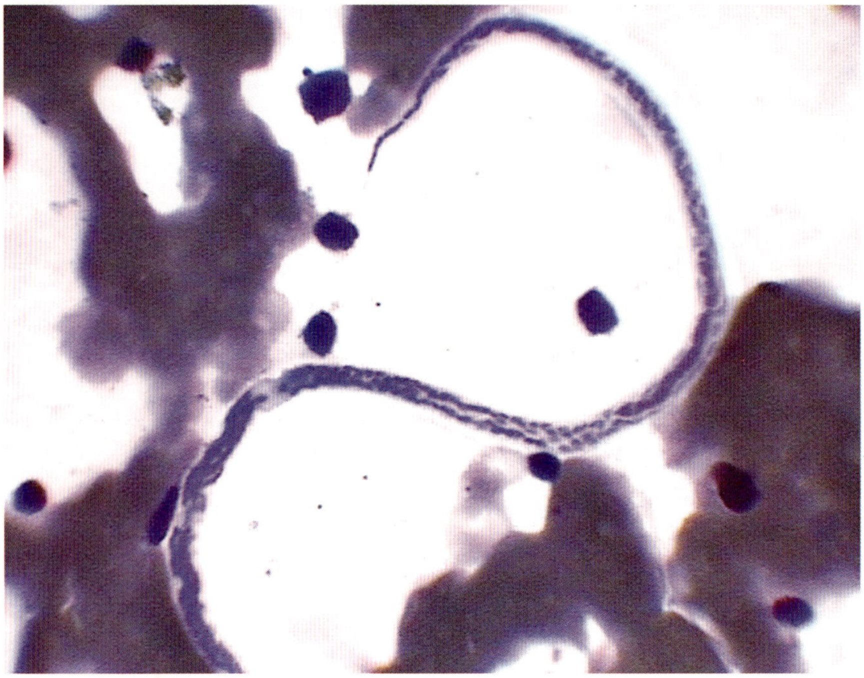

Fig. 9.12: Peripheral smear showing microfilaria

TUBERCULOSIS

In some cases of PUO, epithelioid cell granulomas may be seen in bone marrow. If necrosis is present in these it is more suggestive of tubercular etiology. This may be confirmed by demonstration of acid-fast bacilli (Fig. 9.13).

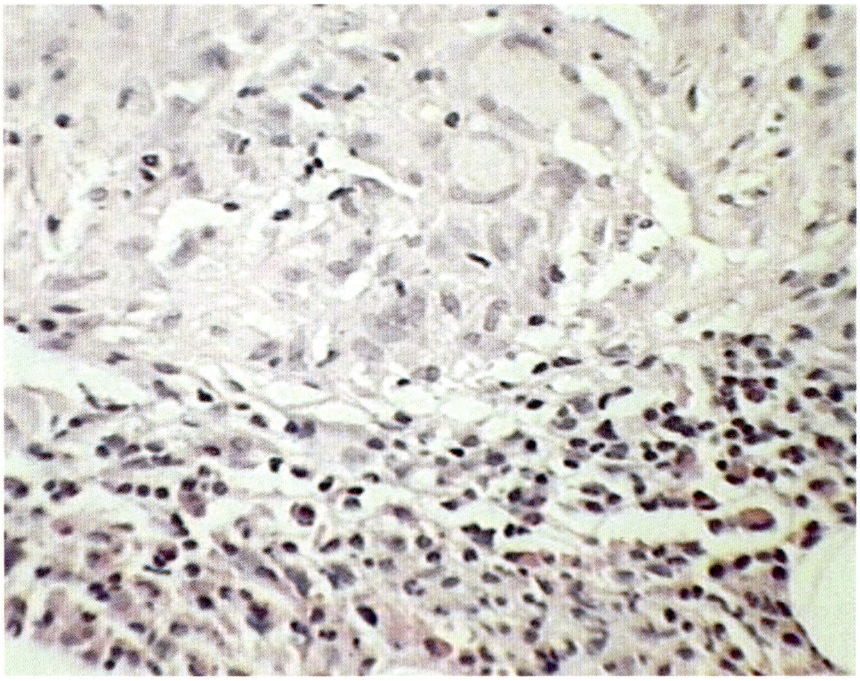

Fig. 9.13: Bone marrow showing a granuloma along with normal hematopoietic elements

Chapter 10

Stem Cell Transplant

CHAPTER OVERVIEW

- Hematopoietic stem cell transplant
- Causes of marrow transplant failure
- Post-transplant MDS

Clinical indications for stem cell transplantation have increased steadily over the past several decades. Most transplant regimens include myeloablation to create space and growth factors for bone marrow regeneration. For peripheral blood stem cell transplantation, additional growth factor is given to donor to mobilize stem cells. The bone marrow aspiration and biopsy are essential in evaluating patients for the above effects. Growth factors result in leukocytosis with a shift to the left in the peripheral blood (Figs 10.1A and B). In the bone marrow, it is associated with myeloid preponderance, prominent granules in myeloid cells and transient increase in promyelocyte cells and blasts. However, these promyelocytes have unilobed nucleus unlike that of APML.

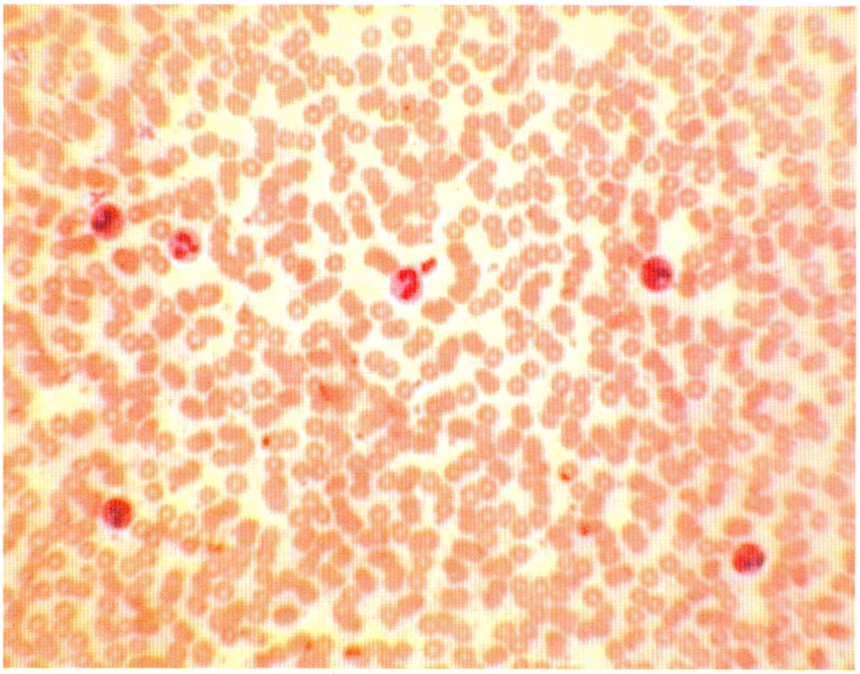

Fig. 10.1A

The morphologic features identified in the bone marrow in early period following transplantation consist of sequential features of cellular death wherein there is massive bone marrow damage with proteinaceous debris. Hypocellularity, fibrinoid necrosis, stromal edema and increased reticulin fibers in the bone marrow are noted during this period (Fig. 10.2).

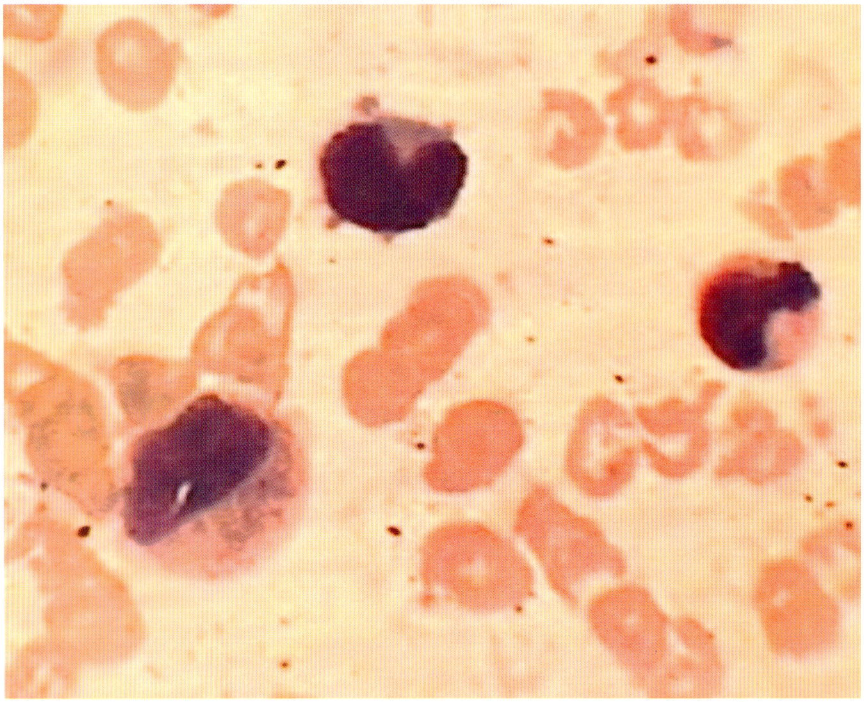

Fig. 10.1B

Figs 10.1A and B: Peripheral smear following G-CSF administration showing leukocytosis with a shift to the left

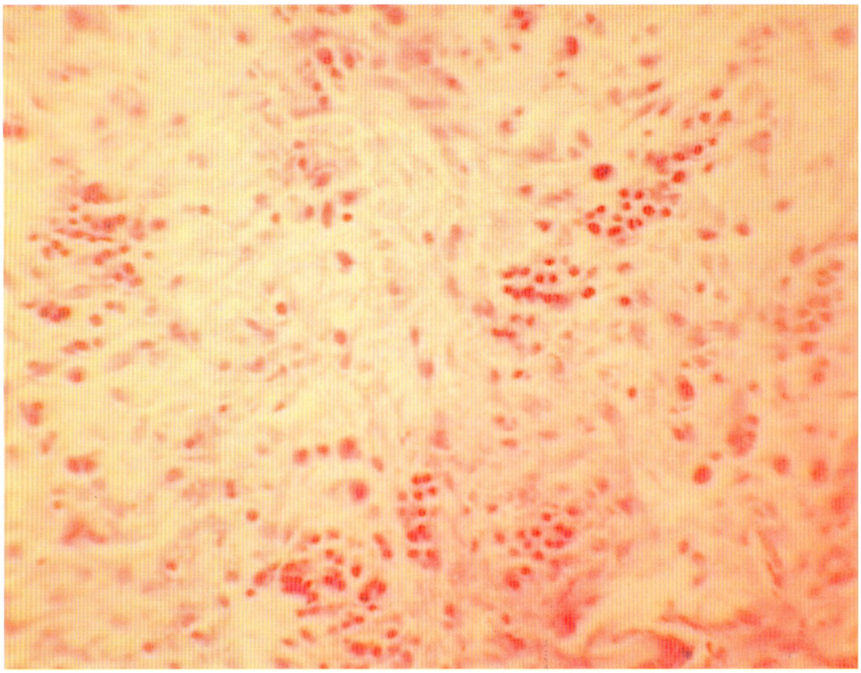

Fig. 10.2: Bone marrow (BM) biopsy following bone marrow transplantation (BMT) showing fibrinoid necrosis and marked stromal edema

Earliest regenerative features in bone marrow occur 7 to 14 days after transplantation and essentially include appearance of non-paratrabecular monotypic erythroid colonies followed by myeloid colonies and finally by megakaryocytic recovery (Fig. 10.3). Absence of monotypic myeloid colonies indicates failure of engraftment.

By day 14 to 21 post-transplant, the colonies become larger and consist of several lineages (Fig. 10.4). Dysmyelopoiesis becomes evident. Neutrophil recovery occurs by day 21, whereas platelet recovery occurs by day 25 to 30. Bone marrow cellularity returns to half its normal level by day 21. Blasts persistence at this time indicates relapse. However, it is important to differentiate blasts from hematogones which may also be seen.

Some patients experience delayed engraftment causes of which may be a T-cell depleted in marrow, extensive prior chemotherapy, ABO mismatched transplant, partially matched HLA or underlying BM fibrosis.

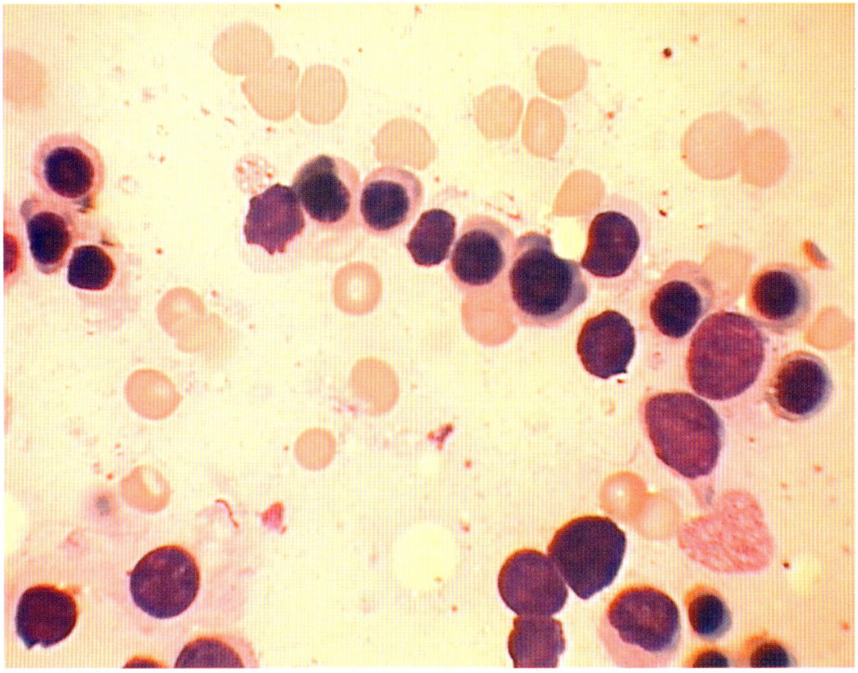

Fig. 10.3: BM aspirate 7 days after BMT showing colonies of erythroid regeneration

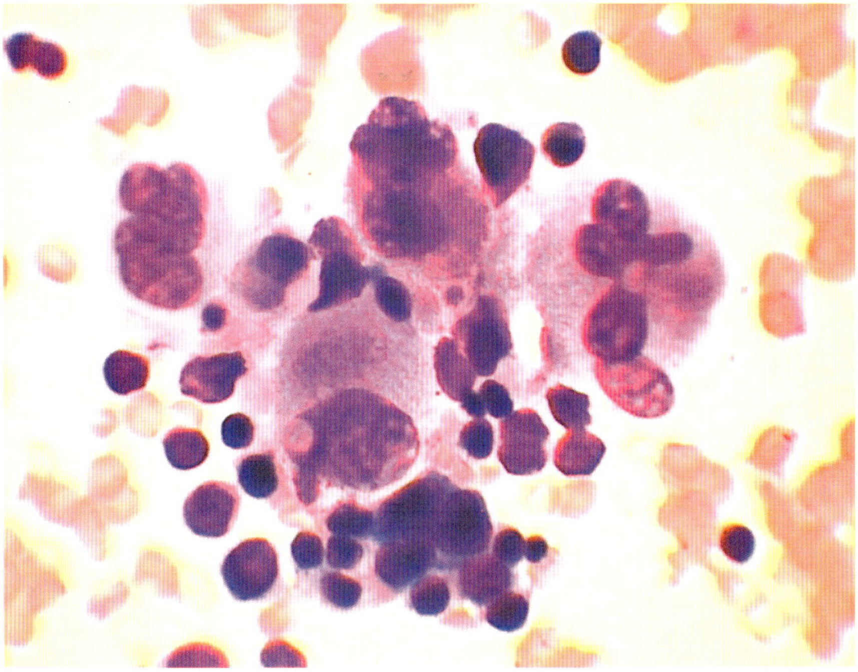

Fig. 10.4: BM aspirate 21 days after BMT showing colonies of megakaryocytes regeneration and dysmegakaryopoiesis

CAUSES OF MARROW TRANSPLANTATION FAILURE

- Possible graft rejection
- Drug toxicity due to drugs like methotrexate, acyclovir
- Viral infections due to CMV, HSV6
- Post-transplant lymphoproliferative disorders.

POST-TRANSPLANT MDS

This is suspected when declining cell counts are seen after day 28, bone marrow shows persistent hypocellularity, fat necrosis, increased histiocytes, plasmacytosis, atypical lymphocytes and absence of hematopoietic regeneration.

Incidentally, presence of atypical lymphocytes may suggest post-transplant viral infections and lymphoproliferative disorders. It is thus essential to monitor the post transplant patients with absolute neutrophil count (ANC) and reticulocyte count for evidence of engraftment and also look for blasts for relapse of leukemia.

INDEX

Page numbers followed by *f* refer to figures and *t* refer to tables.

T

U

V

W

Z